Joe D'Ambrosio

Developmental Dyslexia

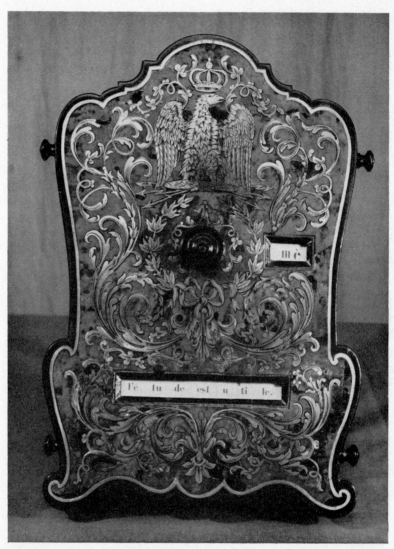

A Second Empire " reading machine " constructed in buhl and vermilion lacquer, measuring 16 × 11 × 2½ inches, decorated with the imperial badge of Napoleon III. This was used by Prince Louis-Napoleon, under the supervision of his tutor M. Augustin Filon.

Frontispiece

Developmental Dyslexia

Macdonald Critchley

Senior Neurologist King's College Hospital, London
Senior Physician National Hospital, Queen Square, London

William Heinemann Medical Books Limited
London

First published 1964

© by Macdonald Critchley 1964 *All rights reserved*

Contents

Introduction

The "discovery" of congenital word-blindness just over 65 years ago was a notable event in medical taxonomy. For the next few decades a series of important contributions betray the interest which this idea had aroused in medical circles, first in Great Britain, then in Europe and later still in North America. Despite changes in terminology, the attitudes towards this disability became firmly established. Of late, however, the situation has changed. The word "congenital word-blindness" was now dropped out of scientific literature in favour of "developmental, or specific dyslexia". The problem began to show signs of ceasing to be regarded as a medical issue at all, while other disciplines, such as pedagogy and psychology, assumed a more active and even aggressive role.

The results of this changed orientation in thinking were both unexpected and unfortunate. When neurologists demarcated "congenital word-blindness" as an entity, they did not for a moment intend to embrace the whole community of illiterates, semi-illiterates, poor readers, slow readers, retarded readers, bad spellers, or reluctant writers. That was a problem which lay outside their sphere of influence, and furthermore only remotely concerned the distinctive cases of constitutional disability in which they as neurologists were interested.

A number of educational psychologists both in this country and in the U.S.A. began to enter the scene, only to obscure the issue at times. Many of these—though certainly not all—regarded the problem of difficulty in learning to read as forming what they called a "continuum": something which ranged from intellectual inadequacy at one end of the scale, to neurosis at the other. This latter, it was alleged, may be the product of such unpropitious environmental factors as broken homes, drunken parents, teacher-pupil hostility, absenteeism, and so on. Many educationalists appear sceptical as to whether developmental dyslexia occurs at all; some go further and proclaim outright that it is a myth. Others say that it might exist, but they have never seen it: or, that they are familiar enough with it, but that it is a psychologically determined illness: or else a manifestation of mental defect: or perhaps the result of starting a child's reading lessons too early; or too late; or of employing wrong techniques: or else it is the price we pay in England for our illogical spelling. So the blame has fallen upon one scapegoat after another, the teacher, the parents, and the child. Even among medical writers there has also been some confused thinking on occasions, for it has been hinted that dyslexia might have something to do with birth trauma: or even with the mother having had more children than was good for her.

The practical upshot of all these muddled ideas of multiple aetiology has been an unfortunate lack of any consistent policy to help the majority of these unhappy victims of dyslexia.

Another instance of illogical argument has been that dyslexia does not exist: or if it does, it is incurable. Neurologists, most of whom would probably agree in believing that there is such an entity as dyslexia, certainly do not support any attitude of educational nihilism. On the contrary, in the recent renewal of interest in this problem, neurologists have been in the forefront in urging an official recognition of dyslexia, and in pleading for skilled screening of the cases, and for appropriate intense and sympathetic tuition of the victims at the hands of specially trained experts.

The lack of serious effort to assist these cases has led to an understandable demand upon the part of parents that some positive action is overdue and that delay can no longer be tolerated. As has happened before, the stimulus for research and treatment in a baffling medical condition has come from interested lay enterprise. Philanthropic organisations like the Orton Society, and the Invalid Children's Aid Association are now intervening in a commendable fashion, and offer a hopeful prospect for the future.

It is for reasons such as these that the subject of developmental dyslexia is topical and even pressing. Consequently it was considered appropriate to expand the Doyne Memorial Lecture for 1961 upon the subject of " Inborn Reading Disorders of Central Origin," so as to constitute the scaffolding of this present monograph.

The chapters which follow seek to trace the growth of our knowledge of this condition, and to describe the conflicting ideas as to nature and causation. Just how these dyslexic children should be taught is an important question which has been deliberately avoided, for this is a technical problem in educational science which lies outside the competency of a neurologist.

A fairly comprehensive bibliography has been prepared, in the belief that even if neurological hypotheses should prove unacceptable to the reader, a ready assistance with the literature might be rewarding.

The author would particularly like to acknowledge the co-operation which he has received in Copenhagen from Doctor Knud Hermann at the Wordblind Institute, and for acquainting him with the problem of dyslexia in Denmark both today and in the historical past.

Lastly, through the kindness of the Editor of the *Evening News*, I am permitted to make a verbatim quotation of a piece of anonymous fine writing which appeared in a leading article on August 9th, 1926:

The Case of the Unlettered.

" 'Although sharp at all other things,' the boy could not read. He was thirteen years old: at thirteen years a boy's reading lessons should be over and done. Yet he could not read: or, if he might read at all, it was only such words as 'cat' and 'rat'.

"Therefore he died, which seems heavy punishment for being dull at his reading. The tramway which runs on Southend Pier is an electric tramway. It is fenced about with railings. What are railings that they should keep a boy from climbing over them? But, besides the railings, there were placards warning all who should approach of the dangers of the live rail.

"If the boy could have read the placards he would not have climbed the railing. But the placards told him nothing, he being able to spell out only the simplest words. So he climbed and took his death from the current.

"The world is like that, a perilous world for those who cannot learn to read. It must be so. We cannot fence every peril so that the unlettered may take no harm from it. There is free and compulsory education: at least everybody has his chance of learning his lessons in school. The world's business is ordered on the understanding that everybody can at least spell out words.

"We walk in obedience to the written word. All about us are boards and placards, telling us to do this thing or to keep from doing that other thing. Keep to the Right, we are bidden, or else we are to Keep to the Left. By this stairway we are to descend to enter the train that goes Westward: by that we go to the Eastward train. Way Out and Way In; Private; Trespassers will be Prosecuted; Pit Entrance; the street's name and the name of the railway station—all of these things are cried out to us by that wonderful device of letters, a babble of voices which make no sound.

"It is hard for us to understand the case of those to whom these many signs and warnings say nothing. They must move as though bewildered, as though they were blind and deaf. No warning touches them, not even that of the board which, like the board of the Southend tramway, cries Danger and Beware.

"Yet they go about their business in that darkness, in that silence. In some fashion they move, keeping shyly beside us lettered folk. Last month one of them sat near to me in a carriage of the underground railway. He asked me how many stations lay between us and the Monument station. I told him that we were not yet near the Monument, but that he was in the right train. But this was not enough: he must needs tell me that he could not read so much as a station's name.

"He seemed a man of sound wits. I dare say that, like the boy killed on Southend pier, this man was 'sharp at all other things'. He wore a coat as good as mine and had the air of one who prospered in the world. But when he told me suddenly that he could not read, I was shocked to hear him: it was as though he had revealed some deformity to me. Indeed I should have looked less curiously at a legless man.

"There he was, in a town all noisy with letters and words, in a carriage full of men reading the news of the world in their news-paper, in a London full of printed stuff, of boards and placards each giving its tidings. Yet he was travelling like a blind man, asking his way, asking help as he went. Another must expound to him the meaning of the plates with the word *Monument* painted on them. Then he would get out of the train and look cunningly to see by which of the staircases men were mounting to the street, for the words Way Out tell him naught. In the course of the day he must have asked many questions and told many men that he could not read.

"When you consider what pains he would be at daily, it would seem easier for him to learn the art of reading than to ask so many questions. For by his speech I took him for a fellow Londoner. On the uplands a man may plough and sow, year in and year out, without ever troubling himself to know the word 'cat' from the word 'rat'. In London the unlettered man must live as one maimed and helpless. But I take it that this poor fellow was one of those whom no teacher might teach to read.

"Indeed I think that there are many such. There are degrees in their ignorance. The man in the train told me that he could read no word. The boy at Southend could read 'cat' and 'rat', although the warning words of the board could not warn him. There are others who can, by setting their wits at it, slowly spell out a sentence, although they do not put themselves willingly to such a task. But none of these can read as we read, to whom the print of whole sentences, of whole paragraphs, speaks at once as we glance at them.

"Nature may have given them good brains and clear wits. Your unlettered man need not be fool nor idiot: it is enough to say that there is some blind spot within his head, some flaw that will ever keep him from reading and writing, from all things that go with reading and writing. Sometimes the labour of the teacher will teach him something of these matters. But he will surely lapse when the teacher shall have done with him; then he will read no more, forgetting all that ever he learned.

"For such as he is, the days of school-time must be long days and weary days. I will not say that all the time is mis-spent: life nowadays is safer for the boy who can read the warning board, although painfully. But the case of the boy who could read only 'cat' and 'rat', although he was 'sharp at other things', should have its lesson for those who are taken by the strong delusion that we may see a world of book-learned men and women if we will spend the money handsomely. For it is not so: there will always be those who cannot get beyond 'cat' and 'rat', even some who cannot get so far."

Chapter I
The aphasiological context

The current neurological conception of a specific and constitutional type of difficulty in learning to interpret printed symbols, took origin from a background of acquired brain disease, out of a process of analogy. Almost as long as aphasia had become recognised, neurology has traditionally taught that in some cases of acquired speech-loss the patient, in conspicuous fashion, may lose his capacity of attaching "meaning" to printed or written verbal symbols. This particular defect is ordinarily termed "alexia" or "dyslexia". The traditional definition advanced by Bateman in 1890 may be quoted: "a form of verbal amnesia in which the patient has lost the memory of the conventional meaning of graphic symbols".

The first evidences of the recognition of such a disability are not easy to trace. The mystical writings of St. Teresa of Jesus (1515–82) mention how during her states of ecstasy words and letters would lose their meaning. Johan Schmidt (1624–90) was, according to A. L. Benton, one of the first physicians clearly to describe the loss of an ability to read. The retrospective personal account written by Professor Lordat of Montpelier in 1843 after his recovery from a speech disorder in 1825 affords a vivid description of his failure to make sense out of printed symbols. "Whilst retaining the memory of the significane of words heard"—so he explained—"I had lost that of their visible signs. Syntax had disappeared along with words; the alphabet alone was left to me, but the function of the letters for the formation of words was a study yet to be made. When I wished to glance over the book which I was reading when my malady overcame me, I found it impossible to read the title. I shall not speak to you of my despair, you can imagine it. I had to spell out slowly most of the words, and I can tell you by the way how much I realised the absurdity of the spelling of our language. After several weeks of profound sadness and resignation, I discovered whilst looking from a distance at the back of one of the volumes in my library, that I was reading accurately the title 'Hippocratis Opera'. This discovery caused me to shed tears of joy."

Other instances of acquired aphasia in which the patient became unable to comprehend printed and written texts, were briefly described by Forbes Winslow (1861); Falret (1864); Peter (1865); and Schmidt (1871). Broadbent in 1872 was an important pioneer in this subject. He described the case of a man who took a friend who had been knocked down in the street, to the Casualty department of St. Mary's Hospital. The porter noticed that the man could not express himself very well and recommended him to the out-patient department. On

1

presenting himself, he pointed to some printed matter on the wall and said, "I can see them, but cannot understand". He had had a slight stroke a year before, since when—although able to write—he could not recognise printed or written words with the exception of his own surname. Though able to converse pretty well he could never recall the names of objects presented to him. Shortly afterwards he died from another vascular accident. Autopsy revealed two lesions, the older one— regarded by Broadbent as being the more significant—being in the region of the left angular and supramarginal gyri.

Kussmaul is usually credited with being the first in 1877 to isolate an aphasic loss of the ability to read, and he proposed the term "word-blindness". In his own words, " . . . a complete text-blindness may exist, although the power of sight, the intellect, and the powers of speech are intact". Dejerine, in 1892, placed the responsible lesion in the medial and inferior portions of the left occipital lobe, but he also surmised that destruction of the fibres connecting the two occipital lobes, was a significant feature.

Autopsy evidence was forthcoming. The word "dyslexia" was first suggested by Professor Berlin of Stuttgart in 1887 in his monograph "Eine besondere Art der Wortblindheit (Dyslexia)".

As further clinical examples came to be reported, it was found that patients with alexia (or dyslexia) could roughly be divided into two main groups, according to whether the ability to write was retained, or not. Some alexic patients were still able to write even though they could not read back what they had written, unless of course the subject-matter remained fresh in their memory. The comment was often made that they wrote as though their eyes were shut. In contrast with these, were those patients who found themselves at one and the same time alexic and agraphic. The custom grew up of regarding the former as examples of "subcortical word-blindness" and the latter as cases of "cortical word-blindness". For years the propriety of such a schematization remained unchallenged. In like manner the conventional belief in an all-or-nothing state of affairs in aphasia was accepted blindly, while fragmentary, incomplete or inconsistent deficits in reading or writing were glossed over.

Another kind of dichotomy also came about, which looked upon cases of alexia without agraphia as instances of "agnosic alexia", in contrast to the cases of alexia combined with agraphia which were deemed to be cases of "aphasic alexia". The grounds for making a rough distinction of this sort are less open to objection.

Finally there grew up a tendency to speak of cases of "pure" alexia (or word-blindness), implying thereby two conceptions which are of dubious validity. In the first place lies the implication—rather than the explicit statement—that the inability to read is total in extent. Secondly there is entailed the notion that the defect exists in isolated form, without any other disturbance of language. Modern aphasiologists, however, are critical on both scores, and suspect that in the allegedly "pure" cases of acquired alexia, other disorders within the realm of language can always be uncovered, if only the investigation probes deeply enough. Contemporary students of aphasia disapprove, furthermore, of the concept of totality within alexia. An absolute, complete and utter failure to interpret each and every verbal symbol is rarely found, if ever, as an acquired deficit.

Hence it is more correct to regard dyslexia as a variant of aphasia where the most conspicuous features consist in an extreme difficulty in the interpretation of verbal symbols by way of visual channels. This last point needs to be emphasised, for it sometimes happens that an alexic patient, unable to interpret at sight a letter or word, can deduce its meaning by dint of tracing the outlines of the symbol with a finger-tip, or by a deliberate sweep of the gaze over the contours. This adventitious mode of interpretation is often spoken of as "Westphal's manœuvre".

In those rare cases of so-called "visual object agnosia" the patient finds great difficulty in identifying surrounding objects by way of sight. The difficulty also applies to persons and human faces; to pictures and illustrations; and of course to verbal and other graphic symbols. When some restitution of function begins to take place, the patient may more or less regain his powers of identifying objects; or perhaps some single objects out of a medley of surrounding stimuli. Thus it comes about that three-dimensional data are understood at a stage when their two-dimensional representations are still elusive. Later still pictorial stimuli may be grasped, but the comprehension of the meaning of letters and words remains imperfect. This, then, is an asymbolia—a dyslexia occurring as the residual disability in a case of agnosia. Other "parietal" defects also may be revealed by appropriate tests, such as constructional apraxia, Gerstmann syndrome, spatial disorientation, defective recognition and naming of colours, or even a frank homonymous hemianopia. Pötzl has asserted that alexia and colour-agnosia always occur together; although that statement goes too far, an association of these two conditions is certainly common.

Complicated errors of visual perception may sometimes be demonstrated in patients with this "agnosic" type of dyslexia. Thus a patient may assert that the printed matter he is looking at is blurred; or that the symbols merge one into another. Sometimes the patient's halting attempts to identify words or letters are assisted to some extent by the use of a magnifying lens. In other words an element of metamorphopsia of central origin may occur in some of these patients and this can either be responsible for the dyslexia, or at least it can aggravate it.

When discussing alexia, a distinction must also be made between the ability to read aloud with understanding of the text, and the power of silent comprehension. Ordinarily the two defects occur together in cases of dyslexia, but occasionally some measure of dissociation occurs. Thus some patients can grasp more or less the significance of verbal symbols which they gaze at in silence; but when they read aloud, the meaning eludes them although the pronunciation of the component words in the text may be adequate. In others it seems as though the double task of reading aloud and of comprehending is one which is beyond the patients' competency. To this unusual phenomenon Joffroy proposed the term "psycholexia".

Of a rather different order is the case quoted by Bastian* where a printed text on being read aloud became a meaningless jargon, capable none the less of being articulated. This same passage has been incorporated by Aldous Huxley within one of his writings, not without certain light-hearted embellishments which certainly do not detract from the narrative, though they do not add to its scientific import. This is how Huxley retailed it:

"Philip was dining alone. In front of his plate half a bottle of claret and the water jug propped up an open volume. He read between the mouthfuls, as he masticated. The book was Bastian's *On the Brain*. Not very up-to-date, perhaps, but the best he could find in his father's library to keep him amused in the train. Halfway through the fish, he came upon the case of the Irish gentleman who had suffered from paraphasia, and was so much struck by it that he pushed aside his plate and, taking out his pocket book, made a note of it at once. The physician had asked the patient to read aloud a paragraph from the statutes of Trinity College, Dublin. 'It shall be in the power of the College to examine or not examine every Licentiate, previous to his admission to a fellowship, as they shall think fit.' What the patient actually read was: 'An the bee-what in the tee-mother of the biothodoodoo, to majoram or that emidrate, eni eni Krastrei, mestreit to ketra lotombreidei, to ra from treido as that kekritest.' Marvellous! Philip said to himself as he copied down the last word. What style! What majestic beauty! The richness and sonority of the opening phrase! '*An the bee-what in the tee-mother of the biothodoodoo.*' He repeated it to himself. 'I shall print it on the title page of my next novel,' he wrote in his notebook. 'The epigraph, the text of the whole sermon.' Shakespeare only talked about tales told by an idiot. But here was the idiot actually speaking . . . Shakespeareanly, what was more. 'The final word about life', he added in pencil."

*This case-report can be found in Bastian's monograph, "A treatise on Aphasia and other speech disorders", 1898, and refers to case 71, originally described by Dr. Osborne of Dublin. According to Bastian the patient read silently with full understanding, but emitted gibberish as he read aloud. The same case was also quoted by F. Bateman in the 2nd edition of his work on aphasia (1890).

An even earlier description of a grotesque distortion of a printed text when read aloud by an aphasiac was given by W. Broadbent in *Brain*, 1878–79.

Chapter II

Historical

Such was the background upon which the conception arose of a defect in the art of reading, which is inherent or inborn, and not acquired through disease.

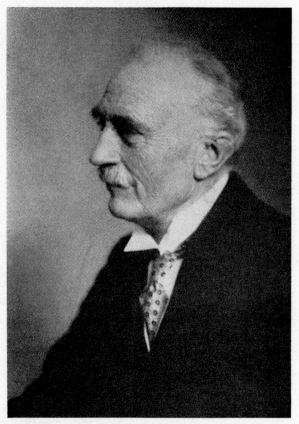

Fig. 1 Dr. W. Pringle Morgan of Seaford, 1863–1934.

In December, 1895, James Hinshelwood, a Glasgow eye surgeon, wrote to the *Lancet* upon the topic of visual memory and word-blindness. This note prompted Dr. Pringle Morgan, a general practitioner in the seaside town of Seaford, where many preparatory schools are located, to describe a paradoxical case which he had seen, of an intel-

ligent boy of 14 who was incapable of learning to read. This was one of
the earliest, and possibly the very first, of cases subsequently to become
known as instances of "congenital word-blindness". Pringle Morgan
sent Hinshelwood a reprint, and in a covering letter wrote: "It was your
paper—may I call it your classical paper?—on word-blindness and
visual memory published in the *Lancet* on 21st December, 1895, which

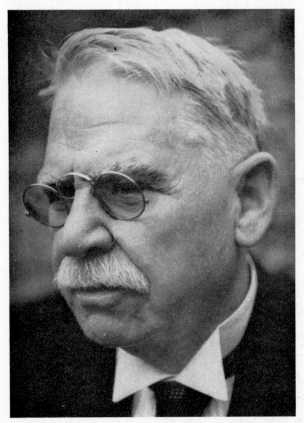

Fig. 2 Dr. James Kerr.

first drew my attention to this subject, and my reason for publishing
this case was that there was no reference anywhere, so far as I knew,
to the possibility of this condition being congenital."

Actually Pringle Morgan had overlooked a note made a few weeks
previously by James Kerr, Medical Officer of Health to the City of
Bradford, and a pioneer in school hygiene. In 1896 Kerr was awarded
the Howard Medal by the Royal Statistical Society for his essay on

"School hygiene, in its mental, moral and physical aspects". Herein we find the following note . . . "But besides the generally dull there are the mentally exceptional, many quite suitable for ordinary school provided the teacher knows their peculiarities. Almost unique cases are found with most *bizarre* defects. Agraphia, for instance, may be unintelligible to a teacher, especially if it occurs, as in one of my cases,

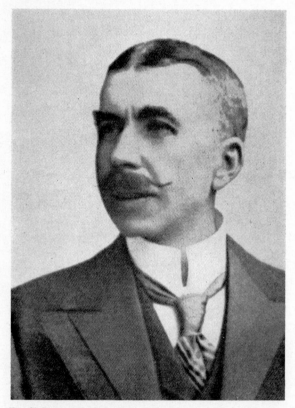

Fig. 3 James Hinshelwood, 1859–1919. Surgeon, Glasgow Eye Infirmary, 1898–1914.

in a boy who can do arithmetic well so long as it involves Arabic numerals only, but writes gibberish in a neat hand for dictation exercise. *A boy with word-blindness who can spell the separate letters, is a trouble . . .* " (Italics not in the original).

Both Berkhan (1885) and Wilbur (1867) have occasionally been cited as pioneers in the history of developmental dyslexia. This is unlikely, for their patients were essentially mental defectives, and an inability to read was merely one aspect of their global disability.

The initiative in the early detection of these cases remained for a time with British observers and especially with ophthalmologists. Among those who became interested were Herbert Fisher, Treacher Collins, Sydney Stephenson, and Robert Walter Doyne. As if piqued by eluding the prize for priority Hinshelwood contributed a series of case-reports in the medical press between 1896 and 1902. In 1900 he issued his monograph upon "Letter, Word, and Mind-Blindness". Reporting two more instances in 1902, Hinshelwood wrote, "I have little doubt that these cases of congenital word-blindness are by no means so rare as the absence of recorded cases would lead us to infer. Their rarity is, I think, accounted for by the fact that when they do occur, they are not recognised. It is a matter of the highest importance to recognise the cause and the true nature of this difficulty in learning to read which is experienced by these children, otherwise they may be harshly treated as imbeciles or incorrigibles, and either neglected or punished for a defect for which they are in no wise responsible."

Outside of Great Britain the syndrome now became recognised and reports came from Lechner in Holland (1903), Wernicke in Buenos Aires (1903) and Peters and by R. Foerster in Germany (1903; 1904). The first American observations were made by Schapringer (1906).

What might be called the early history of this condition was closed by 1917, when Hinshelwood brought out his second monograph entitled "Congenital Word Blindness". This period had been one of description and of identification. Thereafter began a stage of analysis and discussion with a considerable amount of change in orientation. It also ushered in an era of uncertainty.

Owing to many factors, the bulk of research has largely passed from Great Britain to the U.S.A., but even more particularly to the Scandinavian countries. However, within the past year or two there are signs of revival of interest within this country, after a phase of semi-neglect.

Scientific attitudes towards the topic of failure to learn to read have oscillated like a pendulum over the past 60 years. Following Hinshelwood, there grew up the conception of a specific type of inherent aphasia which was at first termed "congenital word-blindness". From the analogy of acquired cases of alexia, a congenital aplasia of one or both angular gyri was visualised, as for example by Fisher (1910). This idea, be it noted, was entirely speculative, no pathological evidence having ever been forthcoming either in its favour or in rebuttal. Indeed, those who imagined some structural brain defect began to find themselves in a minority, and to be outnumbered by those like Apert (1924) and Pötzl (1924) who visualised a developmental delay of functional rather than anatomical nature. Thus there arose gradually the conception of a "maturational lag" to explain the dyslexia.

In 1952 Samuel T. Orton entered the scene. As Director of the Greene County Mental Clinic in Iowa he discovered among a series of retarded children no fewer than 15 who could not read. His first patient was a 16-year-old boy from a junior high school, who had never been able to read. As the boy himself told Dr. Orton: "Mother says there is something funny about me, because you could read anything to me and I'd get it right away, but if I read it myself, I couldn't get it." Orton's interest was aroused and he made the journey to England in order to put the problem before Henry Head, then in retirement. From his close observations of these retarded readers, and from a study of their imperfect efforts at writing and spelling, Orton found other important phenomena. There appeared to exist noteworthy correlations, such as left-handedness or ambidexterity; and a tendency towards reversals when attempting to read and to write—even culminating in frank mirror-reading or mirror-writing. Orton believed that behind all these phenomena there lay a physiological state of ambiguous occipital dominance, a basis largely physiological in nature; a faulty patterning of brain function. For this condition which constituted a kind of graded series, Orton proposed the term "strephosymbolia".

Although this expression has never really gained acceptance, Orton's work broke new ground and directed attention to factors which we now believe may be important in the understanding of delayed ability to read. In the U.S.A. the Orton Society continues to do valuable work in co-ordinating studies upon developmental defects of language and in organising appropriate facilities for teaching such victims.

Later still, the conception of a congenital word-blindness became qualified by opinions of a different sort. What had hitherto been a medical province or responsibility now became invaded by sociologists and educational psychologists. Belatedly, perhaps, they began to probe the much bigger and more complex question of scholastic inadequacy. The illiterate or barely literate population among youngsters gradually became looked upon either as an aspect of general intellectual subnormality ("the mildest grade of imbecility", as Rieger called it), or else as the product of adverse environmental factors. Delayed or diminished powers of learning to read were now regarded—not as a clear-cut entity—but as a non-specific resultant brought about by a diversity of factors. Backwardness in reading even became envisaged more as a problem in sociology. The newer ideas, therefore, were to the effect that cases of inability to read form a spectrum, comprising the intelligent but disturbed child at one extreme, and the dullard at the other, the common feature being failure to learn to read, write and spell. Such psychologists seem either to have overlooked medical views as to the existence of a specific reading-defect, or to have frankly denied its very existence. Thus the very detailed and important studies upon reading-retardation made by Burt, Schonell, Vernon and Monroe, among others, scarcely refer to the existence of a specific and organically determined defect in reading as taught by most neurologists. The multifactorial notion reached its peak when H. M. Robinson (1946) listed some 12 causes, or varieties, of reading-failure.

Among the psychologists who have visualised a smooth transition within the childhood population from normal readers downwards to those with reading handicaps, may be mentioned Meyer, Nørgaard and Torpe (1943), as well as A. J. Gates (1955), H. M. Robinson (1947), M. Monroe and B. Backus (1937), and S. A. Tordrup (1953). Both Hermann and Larsen have independently criticised this conception, and by a close study of the curves which represent the distribution of intelligence levels of schoolchildren have demonstrated a small hump in the region of I.Q. < 45. This was first described by Jaederholm and has since been supported by Pearson, Fraser Roberts, J. C. Smith and E. Strömgren. This hump suggests something more than natural variation, and can fairly be ascribed to the influence of some pathological process. In the context of reading ability this hump is probably to be attributed to the presence of children with developmental dyslexia.

Neurologists, however—while not denying that many cases of failure to learn to read fall outside of their conception of a specific defect—are sceptical about some of these criticisms. Some educationalists have surely been both muddled and opinionated upon this problem; they have also erred by focussing more upon questions of aetiology rather than of cure. Neurologists too have been at fault—not so much in taking up too naïve a standpoint, as in being reluctant to press their views sufficiently. They have allowed psychologists to assert that neurologists regard dyslexics as incurable, and hence take a *non possumus* or nihilistic attitude. This is not really so. Neurologists believe that within the illiterate population there exists a hard core of specific cases which are neither psychologically determined nor yet a facet of mental backwardness. Here we may quote Skydsgaard's definition— "A primary constitutional reading disability which may occur electively". This is a defect in the visual interpretation of verbal symbols— an aphasia-like state: part of an inherent linguistic defect. The victims, if recognised early and handled properly, can be rescued from the limbo of illiteracy, and by appropriate techniques can be taught to read with fair efficiency.

L. Eisenberg's definition is fuller. He would apply the term "specific dyslexia" to a situation in which a child is unable to learn to read with proper facility despite normal intelligence, intact senses, proper instruction, and normal motivation. In this connection the term "specific" really implies an idiopathic condition, that is, one where the cause is unknown. Eisenberg's definition would be improved if for "proper" instruction he substituted the adjective "conventional".

Finally, we can recapitulate the definition advanced by Knud

Hermann: "... a defective capacity for acquiring, at the normal time, a proficiency in reading and writing corresponding to average performance; the deficiency is dependent upon constitutional factors (heredity), is often accompanied by difficulties with other symbols (numbers, musical notation, etc.), it exists in the absence of intellectual defect or of defects of the sense organs which might retard the normal accomplishment of these skills, and in the absence of past or present appreciable inhibitory influences in the internal and external environments."

No neurologist would therefore quarrel violently with Professor Burt when he wrote, "Many striking instances of so-called 'word-blind' children could be cited, who have made rapid and remarkable progress after a few weeks' intensive training at the hands of a psychological specialist" (1950). They would, however, quibble at the adjective "so-called" and they would scarcely imagine that adequate training would be a matter of "a few weeks".

The arguments in favour of the existence of a specific type of developmental dyslexia occurring in the midst of but nosologically apart from the *olla podrida* of bad readers, may be said to rest upon four premises. These comprise: persistence into adulthood; the peculiar and specific nature of the errors in reading and writing; the familial incidence of the defect; and the frequent association with other symbol-defects.

Chapter III
Classification and terminology

By 1917 Hinshelwood thought that already both confusion in thought and loose terminology had developed. He proposed three terms: (1) "congenital dyslexia" for the commonly occurring, mildly backward readers; (2) "congenital alexia" for cases where inability to read was merely part of mental retardation; and (3) "congenital word-blindness" for the well-defined grave cases of pure reading-defect.

This classification may be useful but his terms are unacceptable. Objection was taken both to the adjective "congenital" and also to the expression "word-blind". The latter had already been criticised by Rieger in 1909. Alternative terms like "legasthenia", "word amblyopia" (Clairborne, 1906); "typholexia" (Variot and Lecomte, 1906); "amnesia visualis verbalis" (Witmar, 1907); (Wolff, 1916); "analphabetia partialis" (Engler, 1917); "bradylexia" (Claparède, 1916); "script-blindness" (Strumpell); and "specific reading disability" (Silver and Hagin, 1960) have never caught on. In the United States there has been a tendency to speak of "slow readers" as opposed to "retarded readers", the former being dullards, and the latter normal in intelligence.

Rabinovitch (1954) isolated three groups of poor readers: (1) children of normal intellectual endowment who read badly because of various exogenous factors. Such cases he spoke of as examples of "secondary reading retardation". (2) (a) Children who read badly because of brain damage; and (b) Those endogenous cases without brain damage. These he termed cases of "primary reading retardation". Rabinovitch emphasised that cases of primary and secondary reading retardation also differ in respect of the discrepancies between the items of the Wechsler scale intelligence test. Thus a big discrepancy (averaging 22·1) between the verbal and the performance intelligence quotients suggests a primary reading retardation, while a lesser discrepancy (averaging 8·8) is suggestive of a secondary condition.

Among German authors, Walter (1954) favoured a non-committal term, namely "Angeborene Schreib-Lese-Schwäche" (inborn defect in reading and writing). Nowadays, however, the expression "dyslexia" is most popular, qualified by some such adjective as "constitutional" or "developmental". Most Scandinavian authors speak of "specific" dyslexia. For the less clear-cut cases where the dyslexia occurs alongside other disabilities—linguistic, neurological or psychiatric—some speak of "physiological variants of developmental dyslexia" or, simply, borderline cases.

The term congenital word blindness received a fillip from Bosworth McCready (1926–27) who, while recognising that other terms might be

12

scientifically more exact, considered congenital word blindness "a good robust sounding term, sanctioned by usage of earlier observers". He believed that it was the term which would most likely survive in a medical literature "already encumbered with verbal complexities". For obvious reasons it is the term preferred by various lay bodies, like the Invalid Children's Aid Association, who are endeavouring to fill the gap in our educational system, by providing skilled and individual instruction to dyslexic children. Nevertheless, congenital word-blindness must be looked upon as now outmoded as a scientific term, being largely replaced by the expression "developmental dyslexia".

In this work, the three terms "specific dyslexia", "developmental dyslexia" and "specific developmental dyslexia" will be used interchangeably.

Chapter IV
Linguistic and pedagogic considerations

The inherent complexities of a written language must not be forgotten. The conversion of a spoken language into graphic symbols is at the very least a two-fold problem, for the characters have to cope not only with the phonetic properties of the sound, but also with the problem of meaning. In other words, both phonemics and morphemics must be satisfied.

If the neurological conception as to the constitutional nature of developmental dyslexia be the correct one, then considerations of a linguistic or educational character play a subordinate if not irrelevant part in the aetiology. Naturally these factors, if unpropitious, will still further handicap the dyslexic child who is struggling with the formidable task of coping with verbal symbols.

This "constitutional" view was not always held to be so. Clairborne long ago blamed dyslexia—or "word amblyopia" as he called it—upon the arbitrary pronunciation of the English language, and he seemed to doubt whether this disability ever occurred in those whose mother-tongue was Italian, Spanish or Russian. This attitude is obviously not correct, as experience has abundantly shown. None the less, the fact that English, like Chinese—and to a lesser extent French and Danish—is no logical orthographic language and is not necessarily spelt as it is pronounced, or pronounced as it is written, must erect certain barriers. It is not that dyslexia is unusually common in England, but rather that dyslexics are more readily and more early identified by dint of their failure to master our odd spelling. A patient of Stephenson's was indeed less dyslexic when it came to his Latin exercises than he was with his mother tongue. Though Stephenson ascribed this paradox to the more logical orthography of Latin, many other factors may have been operative, such as for example the technique whereby Latin had been taught.

Without doubt, developmental dyslexia can also occur in countries where the written language is more strictly phonetic, such as Germany, Roumania, Czechoslovakia and Italy. Unfortunately little is known about the incidence of dyslexia in countries where the written language differs fundamentally from the European patterns, and my enquiries as to the possible occurrence of dyslexia in Chinese and Indian pupils have so far been unfruitful. There is an isolated case-report from Japan, where Kuromaru and Okada (1961) referred to a 12-year-old dyslexic boy. More difficulty was experienced in reading the syllabary Kana script than the ideographic Kanji symbols of Chinese origin. It is interesting to recall that in those rare cases of aphasia which have been described in the Japanese, the Kana script seems also to have presented more difficulty than the Kanji. Sally Childs has remarked (1959) that difficulties of a dyslexic kind seem to exist in Arabic-speaking countries owing to the inherent difficulties of their script, but precise details were not given.

The many spelling reforms which have come about in official Norwegian (1907, 1917, 1938) have been blamed as a disturbing factor to dyslexics, greater than in other Scandinavian countries. Again exact information is wanting.

Of particular interest would be a comparison of the incidence of dyslexia in Turkey, where after the revolution there was a compulsory replacement of the right-to-left Arabic script by a left-to-right European mode of writing. A similar problem is likely to arise in China, if reformists succeed in their efforts to impose a Western type of script.

One must also bear in mind the possibility that bilingualism, whether enforced or facultative, may lay an added burden upon poor readers, and so lead to a very early identification of cases of dyslexia. Of Chesni's series of Swiss dyslexics, 22·5% were obligatory bilinguals.

The question must be considered as to whether any of the techniques adopted by those who teach children to read play a part in either helping or handicapping dyslexics. To begin with there is the doubt as to the optimum age at which a child should receive its first lessons in reading, a question which continues to exercise educationalists. In the United Kingdom most children begin to read at 5 and serious reading-lessons start at 6. The age-incidence is about a year later in the U.S.A. L. Bender seems to believe that there is a danger in starting too early to learn to read, and she cited Sweden—where children first attend school at 7—and where some psychologists believe that the late start is responsible for the relatively low incidence of dyslexia. These views are not convincing, and little attention is paid to the role of the mother in teaching the child its letters long before it first attends school. In any event an unduly early or unduly late start upon formal reading lessons could not possibly produce dyslexia, though it might facilitate diagnosis.

Bound up with the problem of when a child should first receive formal instruction in reading is the notion of a state of "reading-readiness". Special tests have been devised with the object of determining whether or not a particular child is ripe for reading lessons. The whole subject is perhaps a little artificial, and is unlikely to assist in the problem of developmental dyslexia unless the test could be shown to lead to a very early diagnosis.

Much discussion has also taken place concerning the possible factor entailed in the various techniques of teaching children to read. Quite apart from any consideration of good spellers as opposed to bad spellers—and the part played by the method of instruction—there is the question whether the newer methods of teaching children to read have led to a more ready recognition of dyslexics. Many have blamed the analytic, look-and-say, "flash" or global systems of teaching—whereby the child learns to identify each word as a whole. Those who hold this view believe that the older synthetic or phonic techniques did not impose such a burden upon dyslexics, who were thereby possibly overlooked for some years. Undoubtedly, sight-reading (as entailed in the analytic systems) presents special difficulties to dyslexics, and also to "slow readers" who are not actually true cases of developmental dyslexia. When this global technique was introduced into American schools in 1926, the progress of ordinary scholars in reading was assisted, but the pupil who for some reason or other was unable to profit by this method, soon became entangled in a web of confusion. Writing in 1937 Orton asserted that he had found three times as many reading-problems in children who had been taught by this look-and-say method. Monroe, too, preferred the old-fashioned phonic approach, saying darkly that it was better to be a slow reader than a non-reader.

Gray—whose primary interest was a crusade against world-wide illiteracy—found it impossible to determine on the evidence available just which was the optimum method of teaching. There is, however, general agreement on one or two scores: (1) that a switch from synthetic to analytic systems of reading assists the quick reader; (2) that it increases the incidence of poor spellers, even among adults; (3) that it imposes a burden upon backward readers, which many may be able eventually to surmount; and (4) that the true developmental dyslexic, stands out conspicuously by reason of his errors and failures, and so leads to readier discovery, with an apparent increase in the incidence of this condition.

A final implication, which will be considered later, is that a dyslexic, once diagnosed, should be taken away from a milieu where the analytic method of teaching is practised, in order to receive special instruction along totally different lines.

Chapter V
Maternal and natal factors in ætiology

That birth injury might constitute a factor in the genesis of dyslexia was first mooted by Fisher in 1910 at a meeting of the Ophthalmological Society of the United Kingdom. Various writers have since suggested that an unrecognised minimal birth injury may express itself in speech retardation, and in later life by serious difficulties in learning to read. Warburg evoked a factor of maternal "Produktionserschöpfung" or weakness from excessive child-bearing or multiparity coupled with heavy manual work during pregnancy. No serious evidence seems to be available, and it is indeed common to find dyslexia in first-born children or in an only child of parents in comfortable social circumstances. Premature infants have been said to develop a higher proportion of reading disabilities, among other defects, than full-term children. The most articulate exponents of a maternal aetiology have been A. A. Kawi and B. Pasamanick, who found that in 16·6% out of a series of 205 children with reading retardation, there had been complications during the mother's pregnancy, like pre-eclampsia, bleeding or hypertension. Of a control group of normal readers, maternal incidents of this kind occurred in only 1·5%. In the authors' view severe brain damage leads to stillbirth, abortion and neo-natal death; while in a descending gradient, lesser traumata conduce to cerebral palsy, epilepsy, and behaviour disorders; whilst the most benign form of brain damage is followed by faulty speech and congenital dyslexia. ... "It would appear that a certain proportion of reading disorders might be added to the continuum of reproductive casualty."

Most neurologists, however, would be reluctant to visualise in developmental dyslexia any focal brain lesion, dysplastic, traumatic or otherwise, despite the analogy of the acquired cases of alexia after brain damage. To do so would be to ignore the important factor of immaturity as applied to chronological age, cortical development, and processes of learning. In all probability the cases of reading retardation which have been observed after brain traumata at birth are of a nature different from the genuine instances of developmental, i.e. specific, dyslexia. This point illustrates the confusion which pervades much of the literature upon the subject of reading retardation and of "congenital word-blindness" alike.

Chapter VI
Clinical manifestations

The neurological conception of developmental dyslexia may therefore be re-stated clearly, before a description is given of the disability itself. Within the heterogeneous community of poor readers (slow readers, retarded readers) there exists a specific syndrome wherein particular difficulty exists in learning the conventional meaning of verbal symbols, and of associating the sound with symbol in appropriate fashion. Such cases are earmarked, it has been said, by their gravity and their purity. They are "grave" in that the difficulty transcends the more common backwardness in reading, and the prognosis is more serious unless some special steps are taken in educational therapy. They are "pure" in that the victims are free from mental defect, serious primary neurotic traits, and all gross neurological deficits. This syndrome of developmental dyslexia is of constitutional and not of environmental origin, and it is often—perhaps even always—genetically determined. It is unlikely to be the product of damage to the brain at birth, even of a minor degree. It is independent of the factor of intelligence, and consequently it may appear in children of normal I.Q. while standing out conspicuously in those who are in the above-average brackets. There is of course no reason why the syndrome should not at times happen to occur in children of subnormal mentality, though diagnosis might then be difficult. Other symbol-systems, e.g. mathematical or musical notation, may or may not be involved as well. The syndrome occurs more often in boys. The difficulty in learning to read is not due to peripheral visual anomalies, but represents a higher level defect—an asymbolia, in other words.

As an asymbolia, the problem in dyslexia lies in the normal "flash" or global identification of a word as a whole, as a symbolic entity. Still further, the dyslexic also experiences a difficulty—though of a lesser degree—in synthesising the word itself out of its component letter-units. Herein lies a two-fold task, comprising first that of interpreting the sound of the word and, secondly, its appropriate meaning.

The syndrome is often said to be "aphasic" in character, in that it represents a facet of defective linguistic attainment. But this is a precarious notion. It is not wise to seek too close an analogy between the non-appearance of a function, and the loss of a function through disease. In any case, the term "aphasia" should not be applied to a failure in the development of a language-modality, but should be reserved for loss or impairment of a mature linguistic endowment. There is still no satisfactory term to stand for a failure of development of language in the growing child. "Alogia" would perhaps be the best pragmatic impression for the idea which is in mind, even though it has occasionally been employed in some other countries in quite another context.

Having set out a descriptive account it would be useful to try and arrive at a definition of developmental dyslexia of workable brevity. Skydsgaard's definition has already been given and may be repeated: "a primary constitutional reading disability which may occur electively". Schilder (1944) laid emphasis upon a deeper aspect of the defect when he put forward the definition: "a primary disturbance of the sound-structure in the written words". Some other writers have attempted to draw up a sort of arithmetical or quantitative definition of dyslexia. Thus it has been looked upon as "a disability in which the reading-age lags behind the mental age by some 20% in spite of two or more years of regular attendance at school, with the usual exposure to both visual and phonic methods; a disability which does not depend upon emotional factors as best as this can be judged. It carries additional connotations in that the disability is a familial trait, and furthermore it is related to mixed dominance."

In the foregoing definition we meet for the first time the term "reading age". This rather suggests that something in the field of symbolic formulation and expression is possible, which might perhaps be correlated with the better known conceptions of "mental age" and "intelligence quotient". Attempts have been made to draw up a series of progressive verbal tests which children at different ages should read correctly. Sometimes the performance is correlated with school grade (as in the U.S.A.) rather than with chronological age. One of the best known Reading Indices in the U.K. is that which is based upon the graduated vocabularies drawn up by Schonell.

From a study of the literature, as well as from the experience of interviewing children who are backward in learning to read, it becomes obvious that we require certain standards of reading texts which will illustrate the hiatus between the child's dyslexia and his chronological and mental ages. There are too many tests offered, rather than too few, and many of them are based upon the American system of school grades and therefore scarcely apply to children elsewhere.

Among the techniques which have recently been favoured by G. Schiffman, are the *Word Recognition Test* and the *Informal Reading Inventory*. The former comprises texts of 15–25 words at each scholastic level, i.e. from the preprimer stage up to and including the tenth grade. Two approaches are adopted, the flash section which measures the sight vocabulary, and the untimed section which demonstrates how well the pupil can employ "word-attack" skills. These are tests of correct pronunciation rather than comprehension. The Informal Reading Inventory (I.R.I.) consists of two sections from each graded basal reader (preprimer up to the ninth grade inclusive). The child reads the words aloud and is then questioned in such a way as to determine whether or not understanding has been achieved. Next the test is repeated after the child has read the test in silence.

M. Monroe (1933) constructed a more elaborate index of reading ability depending upon how the child under observation scored under a battery of diverse reading tests. This author utilised a series of six basic investigations, viz.

(1) *Gray's oral reading paragraphs* of increasing difficulty. Note is made of both the time taken to complete the task, and also the total number of errors. The results are transmuted into a score based upon the child's scholastic grade, which ranges from one to eight.

(2) The *Haggerty Reading Examination*, sigma 1, Test 2, which measures the ability to read silently. The child is required to underline the appropriate answers to questions of increasing difficulty within a given time-limit. The score is given by the number of correct answers, minus the number of incorrect ones. This test is suited to children between the first and fourth school grades.

(3) The *Monroe silent reading examination*. Here a number of paragraphs are followed by a question, and by several suggested words, of which it is necessary to underline the correct one. A time-limit is imposed. The score comprises the number of correct words selected. This list is appropriate for children between the third and eighth grades.

(4) The *Iota word test*, which measures the power of reading isolated words correctly. This test is applicable to children between the first and fifth grades.

(5) The *word discrimination test*. The correct word must be selected from lists of confusing words.

(6) The *Stanford Achievement test* in reading. This is used whenever the child's reading score lies above the norms of any of the previous tests.

Using the foregoing battery, Monroe constructed a "reading index" which takes into account a comparison of the child's composite reading grade with the average chronological, mental and arithmetical grades.*

* For example:
  Chronological age gives a:
        grade replacement of 3·5
        mental age   4·0
        arithmetical grade   3·6
                             ————
        Average =   3·7
  Grade scores on four reading tests were 2·1, 2·5, 1·8, and 2·0, average = 2·1

  Hence the child's reading achievement was $\frac{2·1}{3·7}$ of her expectation, or 0·56, which constitutes the child's Reading Index.

By contrast, one may turn to the relatively simple but practical tests of reading which Hinshelwood employed as a routine procedure. First he would show the young child a picture book containing an illustration of a cat. This the child is required to identify and to name. He is then asked to spell aloud the word "cat". Next he is shown a number of letters of the alphabet which he is required to name. Lastly, he is shown a printed text, and he is instructed to pick out the word "cat" without spelling it aloud, and without moving his lips or hands.

It seems advisable to have at one's disposal two types of reading-tests. In the first place there is scope for a group- or screening-test. This may prove useful in the hands of schoolteachers who might thus be able to identify the backward readers out of a large group of children of the same age. Such a test is the reading section of the California Achievement Test. The backward readers, weeded out in this fashion, will require further testing of a more individual character by way of tests like those employed by Schiffman or Monroe. By such techniques, the putative developmental cases of dyslexia might be sifted from the heterogeneous types of retarded readers. Finally, special neurological and psychological investigation is called for over and above the scholastic tests.

Whatever routine tests be adopted in testing for dyslexia, careful attention must be paid to the speed with which the child reads aloud. Furthermore, the nature and number of mistakes are observed and recorded.

As regards the factor of speed it may be said that the rate of reading is always considerably reduced in the case of dyslexics, whether they are reading silently or aloud. Unfortunately but little information is available as to the reading rates of normal children tested with standard tests. Claparède was indeed so impressed by this factor in dyslexics that he suggested the nosological term "bradylexia". One of his patients, a boy of 10½ years, read a standard text at the rate of 33 words per minute, his performance being marred by numerous errors. The normal reading rate was 120.

E. Bachmann (1927) was particularly interested in this quality of slowness in reading. He instructed six dyslexic and six healthy children to read aloud a series of twenty-nine longish words (i.e. words made up of at least eleven letters). When the reading-time was measured with a stop-watch it was found that the time taken by a dyslexic averaged anything from 1½ to 6 times as long as in the case of normals. Thus a word like "Strassenbahnhaltestelle" (tram-stop) took a normal child 2–4 seconds to read, while a dyslexic of the same age took 39 seconds. "Hitzferein" took 2–4 seconds for a normal, but 115 seconds for a dyslexic. Bachmann indicated the steps taken by the dyslexics in trying to master long and difficult words. Thus, shown the word "Handarbeits-lehrerin" an 11-year-old dyslexic child after:

20 seconds said "Hander . . . "
40   „   „   "Handbar . . . "
60   „   „   "Handbarweisstellerin"
and 90   „   „   "Handarbeitslehrerin".

Another 11-year-old patient was shown the word "Blitzableiter".
After   9 seconds she said "Blitzalbeiter"
„   15   „   „   „   "Blitzahlbeiter"
„   24   „   „   „   "Blitzableiter".

According to Gray, whose primary interest was in international problems of illiteracy rather than individual dyslexia, the reading rates of normal subjects is much superior. Thus when university students were tested, it was found that their rate of silent reading was 5·63 words per second, without undue hurry, but as much as 8·21 at their fastest. When reading aloud the rate ranged from 3·55 to 4·51 words per second. Gray also quoted figures for the reading of Chinese, which, owing to the compactness of the idiograms, can be accomplished even faster. Vertically orientated Chinese writing could be read more quickly than horizontal. The rate of reading varied from 2·8 words per second to 20·7.

Various attempts have been made to classify the errors which a dyslexic child makes when reading aloud. These have been enumerated both by Monroe and by Goldberg, though each employed rather different attitudes towards the data. Among the principal errors may be mentioned:

1. Inability to pronounce an unfamiliar word with a tendency to guess wildly at its phonetic structure.
2. A failure to realise the likenesses and differences between words which are somewhat similar in spelling or in sound, e.g. PUG – BUD; ON – NO.
3. A failure to detect by ear, differences in the sound of words or letters.
4. Difficulty in keeping the correct place while reading.
5. Particular difficulty in switching accurately from the right hand extremity of one line of print to the beginning of the next line at the left. This defect has received particular attention at the hands of Mosse and Daniels, who have described it as a "linear dyslexia".
6. Undue vocalising of sounds while attempting to read silently.
7. Failure to read with sufficient understanding (as checked by such tests as the Monroe silent reading examination).
8. Incorrect pronunciation of vowels, e.g. BAG for BIG.
9. Incorrect pronunciation of consonants, e.g. BOLD for BOLT.
10. Reversals constitute a most important type of errors, and may

entail mirror-opposite letters (according to the typology
employed) Dip and Big. Or the whole word may be reversed,
so that the child may read WAS instead of SAW. Or, again,
short sequences of words may be read the wrong way, as in
the case of "DID HE" for "HE DID".

11. Phonemes may be interpolated incorrectly, as when the child
    reads TRICK instead of TICK.

12. Phonemes may be dropped, especially out of consonantal
    clusters. Thus the child may read TICK instead of TRICK.
    Or whole syllables may be omitted, as when the child reads
    WALK for WALKING.

13. An error of quite different type is seen whenever the child
    substitutes one word for another, e.g. WAS for LIVED. The
    word suggested may be one which is approximate in meaning,
    or one which is metonymous.

14. Words may be repeated in a perseverating fashion, e.g. THE
    CAT THE CAT.

15. Words—inappropriate or otherwise—may be added, e.g.
    "ONCE UPON A TIME THERE WAS" may be read instead
    of "ONCE THERE WAS".

16. One or more words may be omitted altogether, e.g. "A DOG",
    instead of "A FIERCE DOG".

17. An omission of a different sort is seen in the phenomenon
    described by Monroe as a "refusal". Thus the child, attempting
    to read "ONE OF THE MOST INTERESTING" may say
    "ONE OF THE MOST ——" and stick completely over
    the word INTERESTING.

Monroe in her study of children who cannot read, enumerated
ten types of error, viz. faulty vowels or consonants; reversals; addition
or omission of sounds; substitution; repetition; addition or omission of
words; and refusal (including word-aided). Recording these by the
signs V C R A O S Rp Add Om Ra and Tot (for Total) Monroe
constructed charts to indicate a "profile of errors" by dint of Z-scores.*
A single example can be given from a young adult (age not stated)
who reads to a neurologist very like a case of developmental dyslexia.
It must be emphasised, however, that Monroe does not use—and
apparently does not approve—the term "dyslexia" and she referred
to this patient as "a case of severe reading difficulty in an adult of
average intelligence".

* By Z-scores, Monroe refers to the scoring of the number of errors in terms
of standard deviations as they are obtained from T. Kelley's formula,

$$z = \frac{X - M}{6}$$

where X = an individual's score; M = mean; 6 = standard deviation; and z =
standard measure. See T. Kelley, *Statistical Method*, Macmillan, 1923, p. 280.

The role of reversals in the attempts to read and write has often been played down by those who are sceptical as to the existence of dyslexia, and who assert that many normal children exhibit reversals at some time or other during their apprenticeship. But, as J. Money

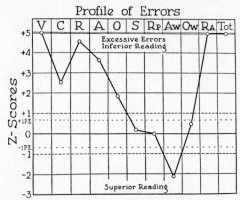

Fig. 4 Reading index 0·41 being case 27 in Monroe's "Children who cannot read".

rightly asserted, the dyslexic individual is not unique in making reversals and translocations, but he is unique in making so many of them and for so long a time. Noesgaard (1943) studied the characters of spelling mistakes perpetrated by normal Danish schoolchildren. His case-material consisted of 300 children aged from 9 to 12, in the 3rd to 6th school years. Hermann compared the errors made by his dyslexics with Noesgaard's findings, as in the following table:

TABLE I

Test Word	Noesgaard % age		Hermann % age	
	Total No. of errors	Total No. of reversals	Total No. of errors	Total No. of reversals
STRAKS (immediately)	11	2·2	99	10
MARTS (March)	21	11	78	26
SLAGS (sort)	24	1·2	81	9
FUGL (bird)	16	10	62	10
KORN (corn)	3·3	0	37	3
ORM (worm)	0·3	0	40	4
VOGN (vehicle)	4·2	3·2	75	30

The greater incidence of reversals among the word-blind is obvious.

When testing dyslexics as to their powers of silent or oral reading it is not infrequently found that the child performs no worse—sometimes indeed a little better—if the book is held upside down. This was so in

Pflugfelder's patient, and it was obvious in many dyslexics in my own series.

To some dyslexics, letters standing in isolation possess little or no identity as units of a verbal sort, but instead they take on concrete non-linguistic properties. Thus to one patient, described by Faust, a capital X suggested a sawing-trestle, a capital Y was a pole support, an S was a traffic sign, a capital P indicated police or else a post-office, a capital U was a rounded arc, a capital L . . . "something that also had to do with police", and G was "an arc with a funny dash in it".

The foregoing accounts of the difficulties in silent comprehension and in the execution of reading aloud bring to the mind of the neurologist many considerations which are familiar to him from his experience of aphasic patients. He recalls that the very term "reading" is an imprecise one, for it entails a whole series of intellectual tasks which vary according to many circumstances, not the least of which is the inherent unfamiliarity of the text. To begin with, it is necessary to distinguish clearly between the problem of reading aloud and that of silent reading. These two activities are in turn capable of a break-down. As was specifically mentioned in the preliminary chapter dealing with aphasic dyslexia, a patient may be able to read aloud with fair phonetic accuracy but with limited comprehension. Or both comprehension and articulation may suffer. These observations hold true in the case of developmental dyslexia just as in aphasiacs.*

Again, the term "silent reading" is ambiguous. Some authors, e.g. Edfeldt (1959), seem to equate silent reading with subvocal reading, i.e. the simultaneous utilisation of silent movement of the lips and other articulatory muscles during the act of scanning a page of text. This is a practice adopted by inexperienced or retarded readers, especially if the text is a difficult one, or if the printed matter is blurred or unclear. This "silent", or better "subvocal", type of reading is probably habitual in cases of developmental dyslexia. Truly silent reading, that is without the intervention of whispers or movements of the lips or glottis, is the

---

* These points require consideration despite the fact that as long ago as 1891 S. Freud emphasized the complexity of the ideas underlying the term "reading". The process of learning to read, he said, is very complicated and entails a frequent shift of the direction of the associations. There are several kinds of reading some of which proceed without understanding. A proof-reader pays special attention to the letters and other symbols the meaning of which may escape him so that a second perusal is needed in order to correct the style. In an interesting novel, on the other hand, misprints are overlooked and it may happen that the reader fails to retain the names of the characters—except perhaps for some meaningless feature, or the recollection that they were long or short, or that they contained an unusual letter such as x or z. Again, during recitation, special attention is paid to the sound impressions of the words and the interval between them: the meaning may be overlooked especially if the reader be fatigued. These, according to Freud, are phenomena of divided attention which are of particular importance, because the understanding of what is read takes place over circuitous routes. Reading aloud is not to be regarded as a different function from reading to oneself, except that it tends to distract attention from the sensory part of the reading process.

hallmark of the experienced and highly skilled reader who is scanning a text wherein both vocabulary and subject-matter lie well within his competency. This last point is important for it suggests that there may be a level of task where even a normal adult is more or less temporarily dyslexic. Such a notion applies forcibly to the patient with an aphasia after an acquired lesion of the brain.

Yet another attitude towards the topic of "reading" and its deficits has been mentioned by Johnson (1961), as quoted by Newbrugh and Kelly (1962). Johnson described three levels of "reading", namely: (1) a *functional* level where the child reads independently; (2) an *instructional* level where the child reads in the classroom; and (3) a *frustrated* level, at which the student misses half or more of the material that he is "reading". The author made the point that the group tests of reading-efficiency measure only the frustrational level, while the individual tests are capable of assessing all three levels.

Again, approaching the topic of "reading" from the standpoint of world literacy, Gray emphasised the graded functional nature of the term. He distinguished an ascending order of interpretation of verbal symbols, viz.: (1) sign reading; (2) gaining information or satisfying curiosity; (3) reading notices or directions; (4) solving problems; (5) thoughtful reaction; and (6) reading for pleasure. These scales are not inapplicable to the dyslexics, who—it may be said—however they have mastered their particular disability, rarely admit to the practice of reading as a form of recreation.

Another point of importance—one with which every neurologist is familiar and where many psychologists are at fault—concerns the characteristic variability of performance of the dyslexic child. The numerous faults in reading which have been enumerated may occur at random in an individual case, being sometimes present but at other times not. A dyslexic child may execute reversals, repetitions, omissions, intrusions and so on at one sitting but not at another. His alleged reading-index may vary from day to day, or from one moment of the day to another: he may fare better with textual subject-matter which interests him, than one which is dull or boring (even though inherently no more difficult). Degrees of distractability, fatigue, and states of bodily health, are variable factors which should be given full attention.

Considerations of this kind convey a certain scepticism about the notion, so favoured by educational psychologists, of reading indices, reading age, educational profiles and the like. Schonell, for example, has spoken of a word recognition age; a comprehension age; a spelling age; multiplication and division ages; a mechanical age; a problem age; a composition age; and so on, in a manner which is foreign to neurological thinking.

When applied to dyslexics, the "educational profiles" as drawn up for example by Monroe, give interesting data, which should, however, be accepted with caution tinged with a little scepticism. A typical example is given in the following charts, where three retarded readers (Monroe does not speak of "dyslexics") are recorded in respect of their performances. (Here O = Oral reading as measured by Gray's Oral Reading test; C = the comprehension of silent reading as determined by either the Haggerty or the Monroe list; WA = word analysis, according to the Iota word test; and WD = word discrimination.)

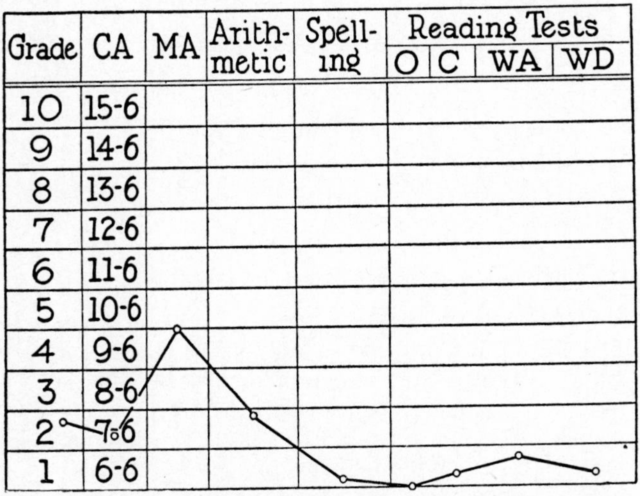

Fig. 5 Educational profile of Monroe's case 3. Reading index 0·41.

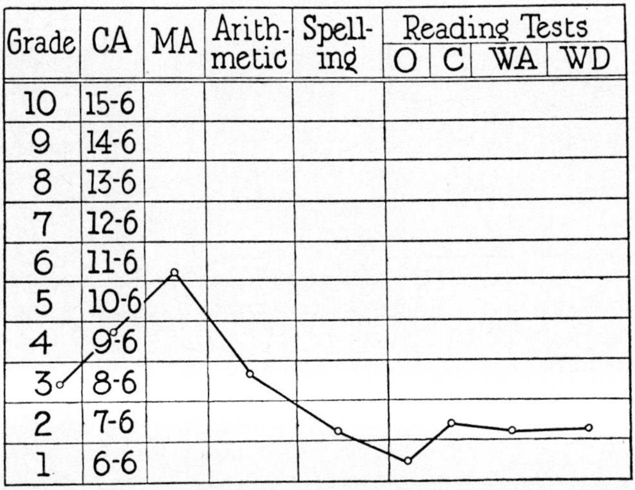

Fig. 6 Educational profile of Monroe's case 4. Reading index 0·50.

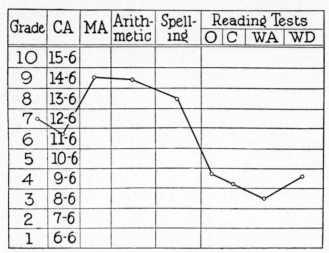

Grade	CA	MA	Arith-metic	Spell-ing	Reading Tests O	C	WA	WD
10	15-6							
9	14-6							
8	13-6							
7	12-6							
6	11-6							
5	10-6							
4	9-6							
3	8-6							
2	7-6							
1	6-6							

Fig. 7 Educational profile of Monroe's case 5. Reading index 0·52.

Monroe's case 3 was a bright little girl of 7 years and 4 months with a mental age of 10 years, and an I.Q. of 135. She had a most engaging manner of distracting attention from her reading-defect. "Let's don't do any reading. I know some arithmetic games that are lots of fun." Whenever a reading task was attempted she displayed considerable emotional tension.

Her 4th case concerned a boy of 9 years and 10 months, with an I.Q. of 130 (on later testing 112). He excelled in mechanical activities. In his own words, "I wish I could learn to read, but I guess I'm too dumb."

Case 5 was a girl aged 11 years and 10 months, with a mental age of 14½ and an I.Q. of 122. Her arithmetical rating was at a superior level. The teachers commented upon her ambition, her social leadership and her general character, even though she admitted to copying other children's book-reports. She read so slowly and with so many mistakes that she could not cope with more than a few pages in an evening.

Less well known than the errors in reading are the disorders of writing, which are always considerable in cases of developmental dyslexia. Berkhan in 1885 made special note of these disabilities in his patients who could not read (but it will be remembered that they were almost certainly mentally retarded). Thus, one child aged 11 years and 2 months wrote *Der Ofen is Hor* (for Der Ofen is hoch). Another wrote *Der Shse mrt Slsl* (for der Schlosser macht Schlussel), *Die Rse st stre* (for die Rosse sind Thiere), and also *Der Vomten lont den Sonne* instead of der Vater lobt den Sohn. Although every child who is dyslexic

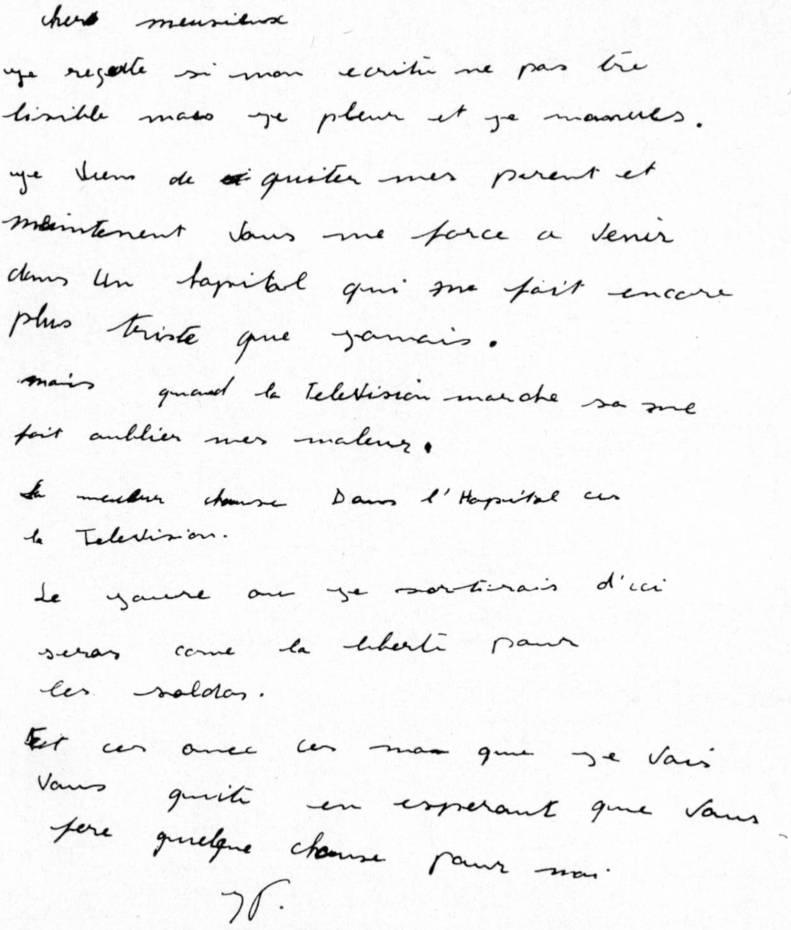

cher monsieur

je regrette si mon écriture ne pas être
lisible mais je pleur et je m'ennuie.

je viens de quitter mes parents et
maintenant on me force a venir
dans un hôpital qui me fait encore
plus triste que jamais.

mais quand la Télévision marche sa me
fait oublier mes malheurs.

la meilleur chose Dans l'Hôpital est
la Télévision.

Le jour où je sortirais d'ici
seras comme la liberté pour
les soldats.

Est ce avec ces mots que je vais
Vous quitter en espérant que Vous
fere quelque chose pour moi.

Fig. 8 Spontaneous writing executed by a French dyslexic boy, aged 15½ years

writes very badly, he can copy printed or cursive texts slavishly and
accurately. He may even be able to transcribe from print to script, or
vice versa. But remarkable errors occur as soon as he writes spon-
taneously or to dictation. Occasionally the difficulties are so great as
to preclude the patient from writing at all. In the case of a "cured"
dyslexic, defective writing and spelling may continue to appear long
into adult life. Where some degree of writing lies within the competency
of a dyslexic, the mistakes are of such a nature as often to make it
possible to diagnose the reading defect from a mere perusal of the script.
The faults are unlike those met with in the case of a dullard, or a poorly
educated person.

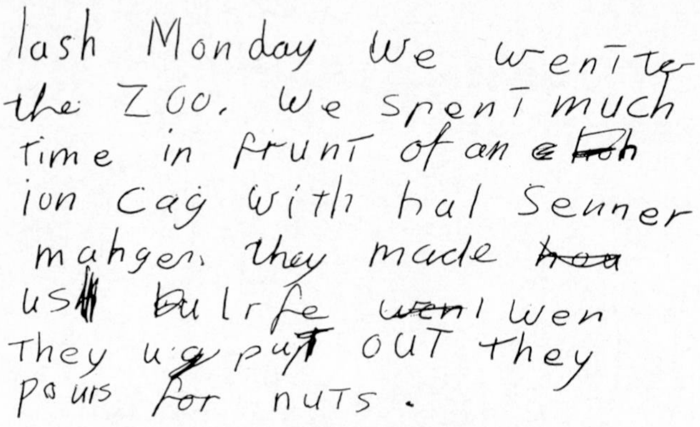

Last Monday we went to the Zoo. We spent much time in front
of an iron cage which held seven monkeys. They made us laugh
when they put out their paws for nuts.

Fig. 9 Writing to dictation. R.G., male aged 11 years. C88584.

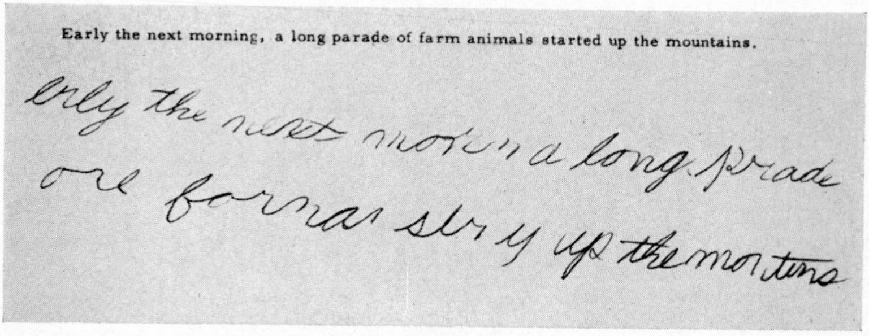

Early the next morning, a long parade of farm animals started up the mountains.

Fig. 10 Writing to dictation. R.S., male aged 13 years.

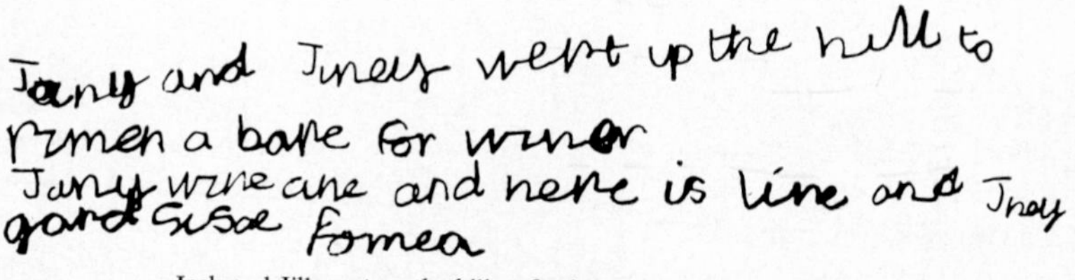

Jack and Jill went up the hill to fetch a pail of water
Jack fell down and broke his crown, and Jill came tumbling after.

Fig. 11 Writing to dictation. J.L., male aged 9 years. C85073.

Writing to dictation:

Fred had five white mice

Fig. 12 Writing to dictation. J.L., male aged 9 years. C85073.

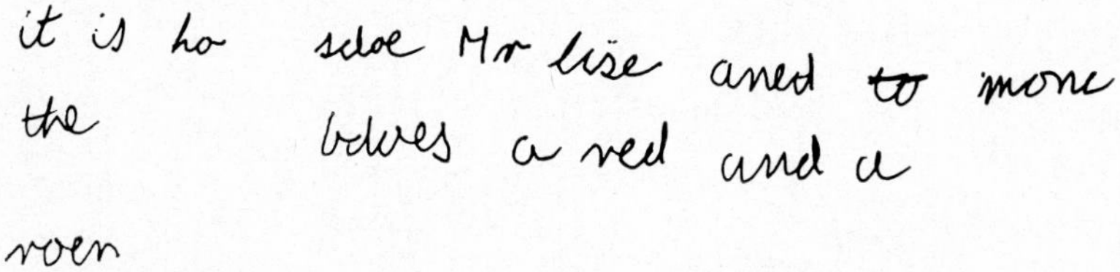

It is hard said Mr. Lemon Hart to make the choice between a red and a yellow rose.

Fig. 13 Writing to dictation. C.C., male aged 11 years. C89235.

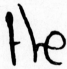

Fig. 14 A fusion of the two consecutive letters " h " and " e " in the word " the ". T.D., male aged 13 years. A5794.

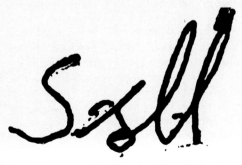

Fig. 15 Fusion of letters; omission of letters; neographisms, illustrated in the word " School ". K.H., male aged 12 years.

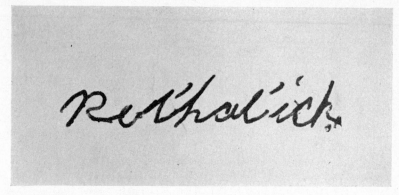

Fig. 16 "Arithmetic", written by M.M., female aged 16 years.

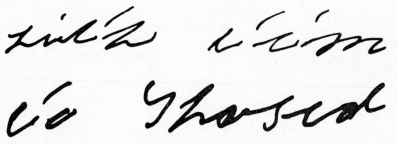

Fig. 17 " Lifetime ", "two thousand " , written by M.M., female, now aged 21 years.

Disorder of writing associated with developmental dyslexia has been noted from the earliest days of this century, but the subject was first specifically ventilated and closely studied by Hermann and Voldby in 1946. Though their observations were made upon Danish children, their findings apply with equal force to English dyslexics.

An overall untidiness of the penmanship is common, but is not essential for occasionally a dyslexic will write in a quite neat fashion with all the errors conspicuously displayed. Among the characteristic defects in writing, the dyslexic may show: malalignment; intrusion of block capitals into the middle of a word; omissions or repetitions of words and letters; rotation of letters; odd punctuation marks; and mis-spellings. Besides the common errors of the ignorant or of the habitual bad speller, unusual and even bizarre mistakes are to be found. Typical faults comprise the partial or complete reversals of groups of letters, so that for the word NOT we may find ONT or TNO, or even TON.

Another characteristic is an unorthodox manner of joining up adjacent letters. Thus the linkages may be either too long or too short;

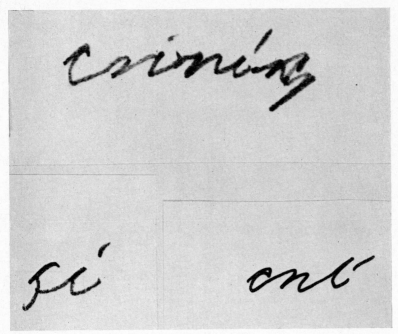

Fig. 18 " Crying ", " if ", " not ", written by M.M., female, now aged 21 years.

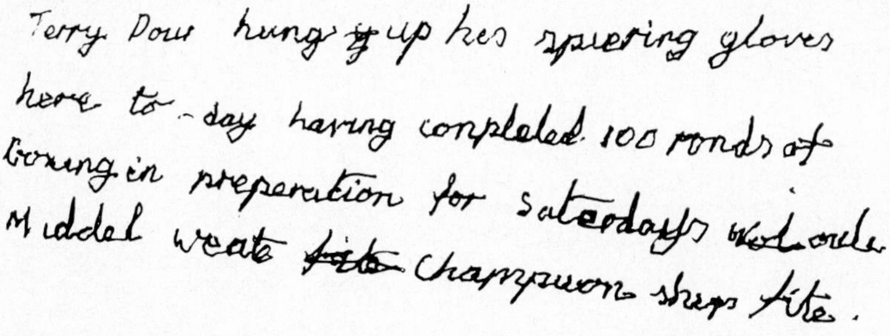

Terry Down hung up his sparring gloves here to-day having completed 100 rounds of boxing in preparation for Saturday's world middleweight championship fight.

Terry Downs hung up his sparring gloves here today having completed
100 rounds of boxing in preparation for Saturday's world middleweight
championship fight.

Fig. 19 Writing to dictation. M.K., male aged 16 years. C78625.

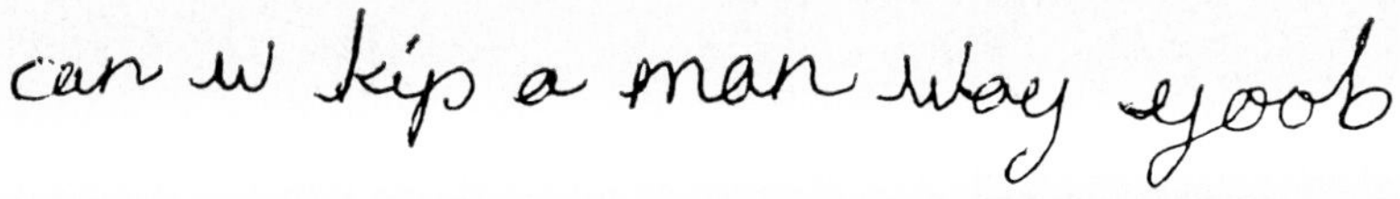

can w kip a man way gyoob

CAN YOU KEEP A MAN WHO WANTS TO GO?

Fig. 20 Writing to dictation. L.G., female aged 21 years. C124680.

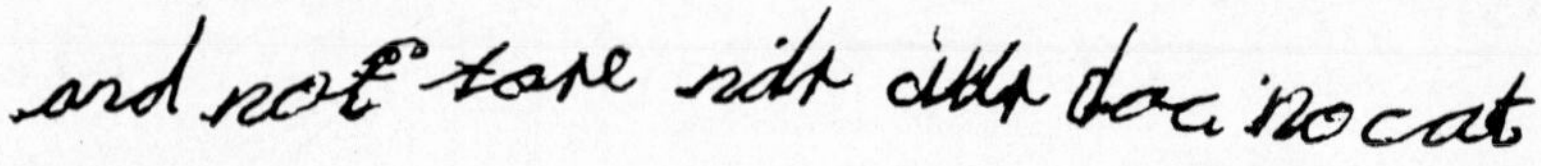

[handwriting: and not tone nitr ditt doc no cat]

Once upon a time there was a man who had a dog
but no cat.

Fig. 21 Writing to dictation. L.D., female aged 12 years. A6660.

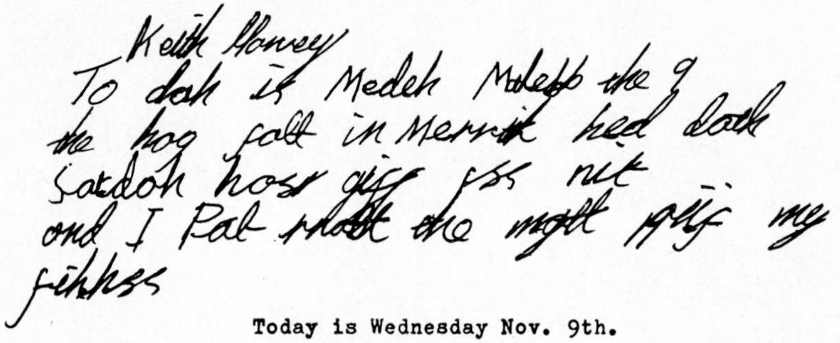

[handwriting: Keith Hansey / To dah it Medeh Molepp the g / the hog fall in Merrit hed doth / Sardoh hoss aff fss nit / ond I Pal plot the moll pluf my / fihhss]

Today is Wednesday Nov. 9th.

They voted in America yesterday.

Saturday was Guy Fawkes' night
and I set off my fireworks around
the mount.

Fig. 22 Writing to dictation. K.H., male aged 12 years. I.Q. (W.I.S.C.): verbal
scale 90; performance 106; full scale 97.

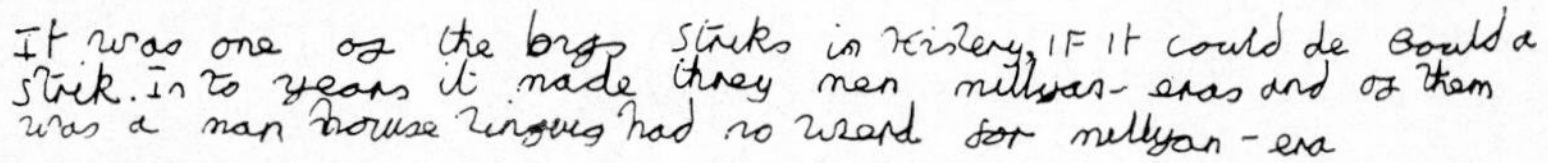

[handwriting: It was one of the brg stuks in Kistery, IF it could de Bould a / Stick. In to years it made they men millyan- eras and of them / was a man house lingus had no word for millyan - era]

It was one of the biggest strikes in history, if it could properly be called a strike.
In two years it made three men millionaires and one of them was a man whose
language had no word for millionaire.

Fig. 23 Writing to dictation. C.E., male aged 11 years 10 months.

or the strokes may intersect (see illustrations). One letter may fuse with
the next to form a strange merger, difficult to identify out of context.
This kind of error is spoken of as a "contamination". Even more typical
are the "neographisms", that is, literal symbols foreign to any accepted
system of typology (see illustrations.)

The spelling mistakes in the writings of dyslexics differ in many
respects from the errors made by normal uneducated subjects or by
dullards. One characteristic stressed by Hermann is the tendency by the
word-blind to employ too few letters, either by telescoping words
together or by omitting letters. Various examples were given by Hermann. The Danish words "ner var" (now was) may be represented by

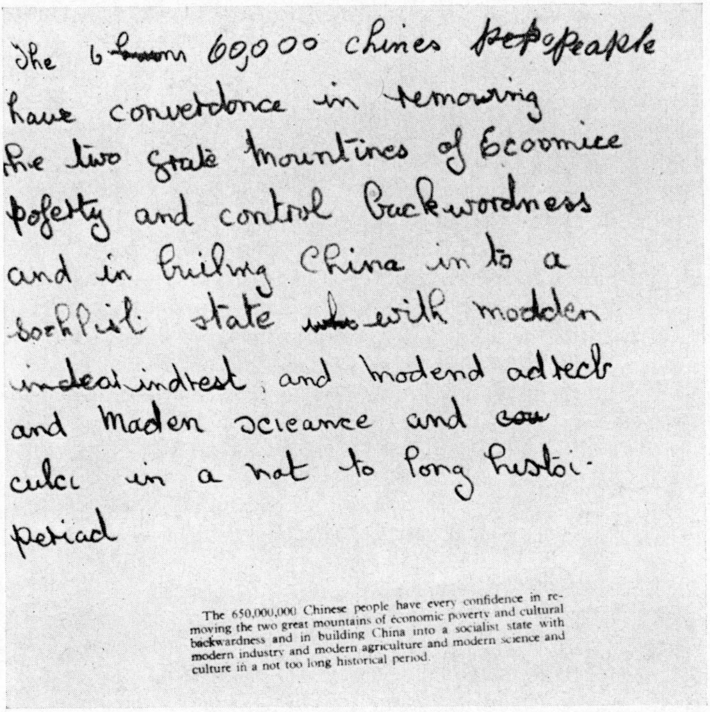
The 6 60,000 chines peaple
have converdonce in temowring
the two grate mountines of Ecoomice
pofesty and control Backwordness
and in builing China in to a
sochlist state with modden
indrest, and modend adtech
and Maden scieance and
culci in a not to long histoi-
periad
The 650,000,000 Chinese people have every confidence in removing the two great mountains of economic poverty and cultural backwardness and in building China into a socialist state with modern industry and modern agriculture and modern science and culture in a not too long historical period.

Fig. 24 Writing to dictation. A.S.K., male aged 41 years. A5440.

"nva"; "to stags" (two sorts) becomes "tostg"; "i naerheden" (in the vicinity) was spelt "inehed". Illing's patient contracted the German sentence "im Hofe steht ein Schneemann" into "imhfeoscheischm". In a Norwegian dyslexic's writing "pa primusen" (on the primus) was rendered "apmisen". As to the letters which are most likely to be dropped Hermann mentioned mute letters and vowels, the general tendency being for the dyslexic to spell, as he writes, phonetically rather than conventionally.

Hermann was of the opinion that the disordered writing of developmental dyslexics shows among other defects, certain apractic characteristics. This is illustrated when the child can spell aloud a word, e.g. C–A–T and then say "cat", but writes it down as "cad". The confusion of T and D is looked upon by Hermann as evidence of ideomotor apraxia. Of course this is not the sole reason for the incorrect transcription of letters. Hermann has been struck by the frequency with which a dyslexic child will proclaim that he has forgotten "what a particular letter looks like" and he consequently writes down a malformed character. This is evidence of an ideational defect. Herein lies the explanation of the various neographisms already referred to, including the contaminations, or fusion of fragments of two adjacent letters.

The foregoing errors are not identical with the mistakes commonly witnessed in patients who have developed an aphasia late in life. It is not altogether correct, therefore, to speak of a "developmental dysgraphia" in this connection, as some have done. The true "dysgraphic" is an adult of at least normal education, who has developed a difficulty in expressing himself on paper as the result of disease. A study of the script will show a breakdown of what had previously been a rapidly executed and highly individual motor-skill with many characteristics, which to a graphologist are personal and specific. Many of these revealing features will still be identifiable, despite the dysgraphia: they may even be exaggerated. The situation is quite different in the case of a developmental dyslexic who is attempting to write. No motor skill has been achieved and no individual peculiarities have developed. The situation is not so much a break-down of a consummate faculty as a failure of accomplishment.

A less well-known defect, but a highly characteristic one, is inability on the part of the dyslexic to "spell in numbers". This is shown by a

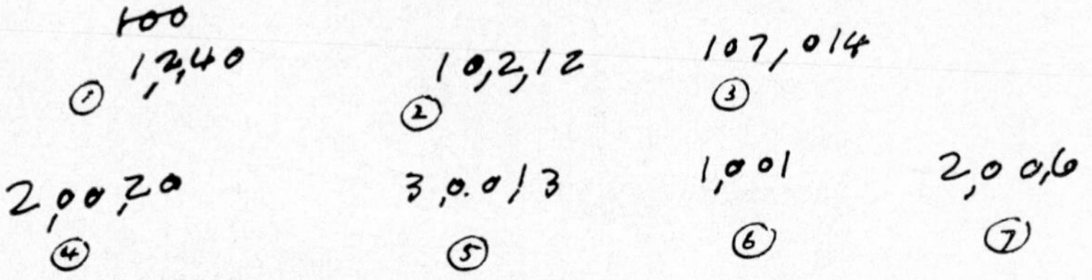

Patient was asked to write down:-
(1) 1,240   (2) 10,212   (3) 107,014
(4) 2,000,020   (5) 3,000,013   (6) 1,001   (7) 200,006

Fig. 25 Dictation of numerals. M.M., female aged 21 years.

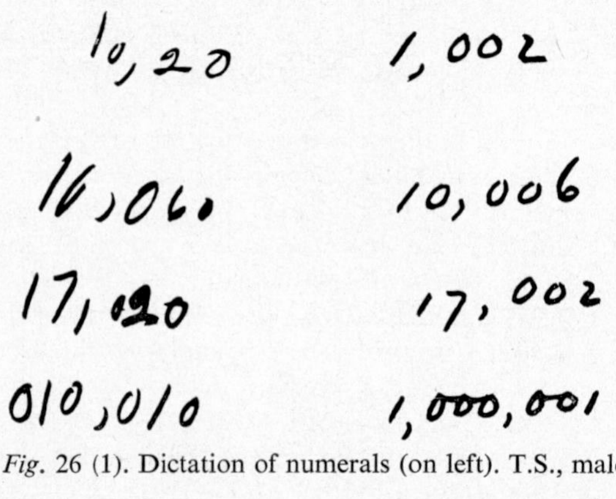

Fig. 26 (1). Dictation of numerals (on left). T.S., male aged 11 years.

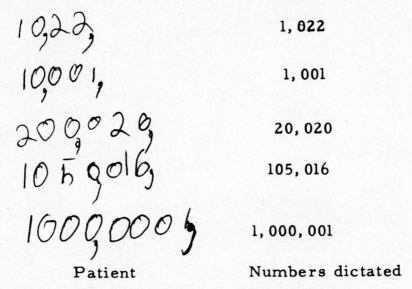

	1, 022
	1, 001
	20, 020
	105, 016
	1, 000, 001
Patient	Numbers dictated

Fig. 26(2) Dictation of numerals. K.C., male aged 10 years. C82100.

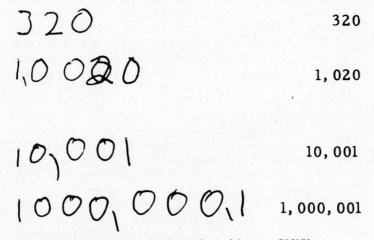

	320
	1, 020
	10, 001
	1, 000, 001

Fig. 27 Dictation of numerals. J.L., male aged 9 years. C85073.

difficulty in setting down on paper to dictation long numbers entailing many digits. There may be too many noughts, or too few. Especial confusion arises over the correct placing of the commas. Thus, told to write down one hundred and forty-six, the dyslexic may put down "100, 46"; for a "million and one" he may write, 1, 00, 01 (see illustra-

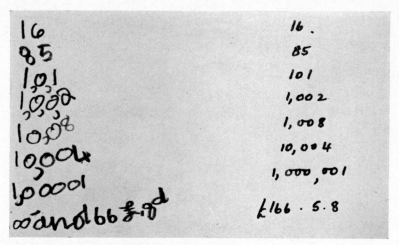

Fig. 28 Dictation of numerals. C.C., male aged 11 years. C89235.

tions). Although an anomaly in numerical spelling was mentioned by Stahli, and also by Faust, it has not yet received the attention which it merits as a common feature in dyslexia. Hermann had also noticed how often a dyslexic will insert extra noughts when directed to write down a number to dictation.

Arithmetical retardation may be associated with developmental dyslexia, but not necessarily so. Indeed, many authors and particularly the earlier ones, have commented upon that paradoxical state of affairs which some of their patients have shown, in being advanced in their arithmetical prowess while grossly defective as to their ability to read. On the other hand, some writers have found that their dyslexic patients are often confused over the recognition of numerical symbols to the detriment of their powers of calculation. When in addition to difficulties in the identification of literal symbols, there also occurs an imperfect recognition of numerals, then a dyscalculia is bound to follow. Difficulties in calculation may be experienced by some word-blind children for a diversity of reasons. Apart from what may be termed "number-blindness" there may exist a higher-level dyscalculia, made up partly at any rate by an inability to visualise numbers or to retain a series of digits in the memory for a sufficient length of time. But in some at least of these cases, "mental arithmetic" is carried out with fair success, even though calculations upon paper are poorly performed. A few observers like Kopp, have, however, commented upon the mathematical skill displayed by some dyslexic patients, who may even become accountants. It is as though they were more at ease upon levels of higher abstraction than with verbal symbols. "They transfer to numbers some of the pleasure others have in words."

A similar inconsistency applies to the artistic abilities of dyslexics. Ordinarily their achievement is to be rated as average, while many of these children seem to be peculiarly inept as regards their drawing. In some cases at least, though certainly not in all, there appears to exist no conception of perspective in their work, and it is tempting to invoke in such cases an inherent defect in spatial thought. But on the other hand some dyslexic children draw well: others indeed have excelled if not in draughtsmanship, then in their use of colour. This state of affairs has been expressly described by L. Bender who reproduced the pictorial art of two of her dyslexic patients, Marcellus and Albert. At an earlier date Kopp, who has already been quoted in association with the arithmetical abilities of dyslexics, had stated that some of these children "take a particular pleasure in a colourful world of fantasy, invest fantastic stories, and do elaborate handicraft work".*

* It is interesting to read a layman's view of the relationship between backwardness in reading and special aptitude in drawing and painting. M. Augustin Filon, who was tutor to the Prince Imperial, only son of the Emperor Napoleon III, found great difficulty in teaching his pupil the elements of reading, writing and spelling. But he was unusually adroit at art-work. Regarding this talent, Filon wrote: " . . . the astonishing gift which characterised the Prince, the memory of contours and colours, was perhaps one of the reasons that made it hard for him to attain a knowledge of spelling. When a word was pronounced to him, he saw in his mind's eye the man or the thing, and not a printed word". (*Memoirs of the Prince Imperial (1856–1879)* by Augustin Filon. Heinemann, London, 1913, p. 46.)
In 1954 a German newspaper carried the story of Jack Taylor, an uneducated, dyslexic Englishman of 24 years who was found to be a talented painter of promise. A successful exhibition of his work was held at the Redfern Gallery. At school he had been quite unable to learn to read.

Chapter VII
Ophthalmological aspects

Developmental dyslexia is independent of errors of refraction; muscle imbalance, and imperfect binocular fusion. This statement is possible despite the correlation noted, or the causal importance claimed, by Betts (1936), Eames (1932–48) and others, between reading-disability and such visual defects as heterophoria, fusion anomalies, field restriction and hypermetropia. No correlation exists between the degree of binocular co-ordination and reading ability (Gruber, 1962). The problem as to whether the perception of visual sense-data is disturbed or not will be discussed more fully later.

Minor upsets in the discrimination of colours, or perhaps merely in their correct naming, have been mentioned by a number of writers, particularly in Germany (e.g. Warburg, 1911; Laubenthal, 1936; Pflugfelder, 1948). In my own cases I have not found such disorders.

The question may be posed whether more subtle ocular examinations might perhaps uncover certain defects, though the problem would still arise as to whether these were the product or the cause of the dyslexia. Thus Lasèvre et al. have been measuring the reaction-time preceding willed movements of the eyes to command in normals and in dyslexics. Certain standards were established, including the observation that the latency of movements to the right differed slightly from that of movements to the left. In dyslexic children not only were all eye-movements slower in initiation, but furthermore the usual difference between right and left ocular deviation was not present.

Of more immediate importance is the question as to the nature of reading movements of the eyes in dyslexics as compared with normals.

The interesting topic of the character of the ocular movements performed by normal persons and others during the act of reading, has been studied by various techniques including photographic, electro-encephalographic and scopographic. Considerable variation has been found to occur from one individual to another, depending upon a diversity of factors such as for example the nature of the reading matter; the length of the lines; the size of the type; and in particular the content of the text and the words entailed. Among the personal factors which seem to be important determinants are age, and more especially the cultural and intellectual status. Ophthalmographic studies may therefore adduce important objective information as to a person's reading efficiency. Such studies take note of the number and duration of pauses (fixations, or "stations du regard"); the number and amplitude of regressions

TEMPS DE RÉACTION OCULO MOTEUR ET DIRECTION DU REGARD

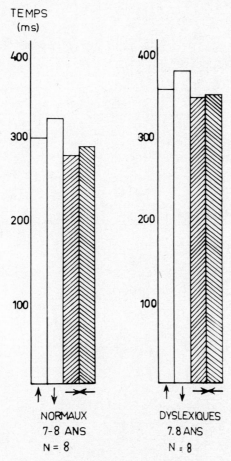

Fig. 29 Measurement of the reaction time preceding willed movements of the eyes up, down, to the right and to the left, in normal children and in dyslexics. (After Lasèvre *et al.*).

(or backward movements of the eyes); the span of words encompassed by each sweep; and the rate of comprehension. Depending upon the character of the eye-movements is the overall rate of reading. Ordinarily a reader absorbs a printed page by identify-

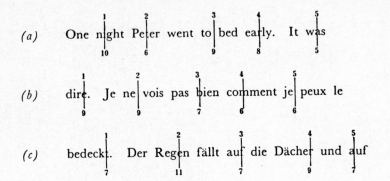

Examples of eye-movement records in three languages: (a) a college student in the United States[3]; (b) an efficient reader of French;[4] (c) a native German reader.[5] In this and the following figure, the vertical lines represent centres of fixations. The numbers above the lines indicate the serial order of fixations; those below indicate duration in thirtieths of a second.

Fig. 30 Records of eye movements during the act of reading (after Gray).

LECTURE ET NIVEAU CULTUREL

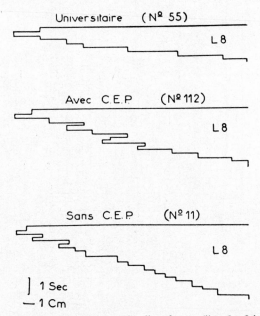

3 exemples de scopogramme d'une même ligne de texte (ligne 8, « Soir de Vendange ») représentatifs de *niveaux culturels différents* : depuis le niveau universitaire jusqu'à celui de sujets sans certificat d'études. En passant par des individus d'un niveau intermédiaire la largeur des plages de lecture croît avec le niveau culturel alors que le nombre de vérifications, le temps de lecture par ligne et la durée des stations diminue parallèlement.

Fig. 31 Records of eye movements during the act of reading in normal subject of three different cultural levels (after Rémond *et al.*).

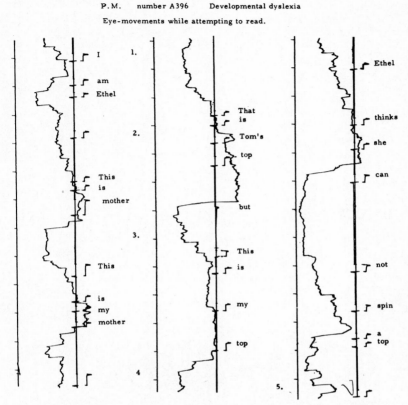

P.M. number A396 Developmental dyslexia

Eye-movements while attempting to read.

Fig. 32 Record of eye movements during the act of attempting to read, in a dyslexic. P.M., aged 31. A396. (Courtesy of Dr. Hallpike.)

ing either single words or phrases; or groups of letters; or perhaps only individual letters at a time, according to the degree of familiarity of the reader with his material; his skill or practice; and the inherent clarity or obscurity of the text. Most adults manage about 300 words per minute. A few gifted readers can cope with 1,000 words per minute, or even more. One young prodigy in E. A. Taylor's series mastered as many as 2,200 words per minute. Most college professors, be it noted, do not read more than 350 or at the most 500 words in a minute. The aptitude improves in rate and in quality with age and education (see Table II), and the reading rate can be deliberately and considerably enhanced by dint of special training techniques.

Ocular movements are naturally altered in certain pathological conditions like hemianopia, the pattern differing according to whether

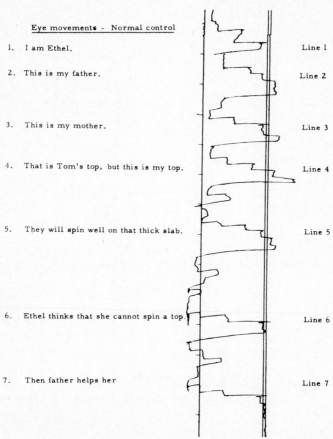

Eye movements - Normal control

1. I am Ethel.   Line 1

2. This is my father.   Line 2

3. This is my mother.   Line 3

4. That is Tom's top, but this is my top.   Line 4

5. They will spin well on that thick slab.   Line 5

6. Ethel thinks that she cannot spin a top.   Line 6

7. Then father helps her   Line 7

Fig. 33 Eye movements during the act of reading the same text as by the patient P.M. (Fig. 32). Normal control. (Courtesy of Dr. Hallpike)

TABLE II. *Measurable Components of the Fundamental Reading Skill*

GRADE LEVEL	1st	2nd	3rd	4th	5th	6th	Jr. HS	HS	College
Fixations per 100 words	240	200	170	136	118	105	95	83	75
Regressions per 100 words	55	45	37	30	26	23	18	15	11
Average span of recognition (in words)	0·42	0·50	0·59	0·73	0·85	0·95	1·05	1·21	1·33
Average duration of fixation (in seconds)	0·33	0·30	0·26	0·24	0·24	0·24	0·24	0·24	0·23
Average rate of comprehension (in words per minute)	75	100	138	180	216	235	255	296	340

Compiled by E. A. Taylor (1957) from over 5,000 eye-movement records.

the homonymous visual loss lies to the right or to the left of the midline. In aphasic patients who have an alexic difficulty in the comprehension of verbal symbols, the movements of the eyes during the act of attempting to read, are necessarily much deranged. This subject has not yet been sufficiently explored for one to be able to analyse and clarify these defects.

It is not surprising to find that unusual ocular movements occur in the case of inherently poor readers, and of developmental dyslexics in particular. Unfortunately the material that has been studied so far is not great. Sometimes it has been asserted that abnormal eye movements are the actual cause of backwardness in learning to read. Hildreth (1936), for example, alleged that "reversals of letter-sequence in perceiving certain words are due to faulty eye movements". P. A. Witty and D. Kopel (1936) stated that left eye dominance, in some cases, results in the eyes moving from right to left during the act of reading, presumably causing difficulty or delay in comprehension. H. L. Mosse and C. R. Daniels (1959), who described a particular defect in the return sweep from the end of one line to the start of the next ("linear dyslexia") went on to assert that anomalies in this manœuvre are responsible for difficulty in comprehension, arising in turn from faulty habits of reading which are psychologically determined.

But arguments of this kind are surely topsy-turvy. Faulty eye movements must be regarded as the outcome of a difficulty in reading, and not its cause. An analogy with the disordered reading movements of the eyes shown by aphasic subjects can be fairly made. A possible exception to this statement may be found in the curious group of cases described by H. F. R. Prechtl and J. C. Stemmer. Out of a series of children with learning difficulties, a distinct neurological sydrome could be identified in 50 cases. These showed habitual clumsiness with choreiform movements. In 96% of such children the eye muscles were similarly affected, leading to disturbances of conjugate movement and difficulty in fixation and reading. It was alleged by Prechtl that the choreiform activity caused both difficulty in mental concentration and also in fixating during the act of reading. Obviously this report bears little or no relationship to the problem of specific developmental dyslexia.

Closely bound up with the subject of eye movements in the act of reading is the question of the rate of identification of verbal symbol units, as studied tachistoscopically.

From his experience of normal subjects Gray was able to assert that at a single short exposure, it is possible to identify four or five unrelated letters, or words made up of four or five times that number of letters. The number of symbols perceived at each exposure depends partly upon the extent to which the material "makes sense". In the recognition of new words, certain letters are perceived more quickly than others, e.g. letters with a distinctive shape, or those which extend above or below the horizontal line. Such letters attract particular attention, and supply clues to the recognition of the word as a whole.

Similar tachistoscopic testing was applied to cases of developmental dyslexia by F. Bachmann (1927). Normal and dyslexic children were shown words both meaningful and meaningless, and words with or without sound-pictures. Exposures were of 0·2 sec., 0·5 sec. and 1 sec., beginning with short words (i.e. of three or four letters) and rising to words composed of so many letters that reading became impossible. His findings caused him surprise. It was found that the limit of readability was reached with the same number of letters in the case of dyslexics and normal children alike. However, the number of letters in the words entailed was small. The rate of reading was found to be diminished in the dyslexics in these tachistoscopic tests, and this applied both to real words and to nonsense words.

Tachistoscopic studies were also carried out by P. Schilder (1944). From close observation of seven subjects he found that difficulty in perception during the ordinary act of reading was usually confined to letters and words rather than numerical symbols. Four-digit numbers were identified, whereas four-letter words were not. Pictures were recognised as a rule and there was no trace of mirror-mistakes. The accuracy of picture recognition contrasted markedly with the difficulties and delays in word-recognition. When verbal symbols were presented tachistoscopically, no increase in the difficulty in recognition resulted. Schilder drew some important conclusions from these data. The situation seemed to be quite unlike what was found in the acquired alexics of adulthood, where the difficulty in perception was a pure optic product. But in the case of the developmental dyslexic (or congenital word-blind, as he said) . . . "the difficulty concerns the inner structure of the word and its sounds. It is an agnostic trouble, not so much concerning the merely optic sphere, but a sphere which is nearer to the intellectual life than the optic perception. It is true that every gnostic function is also an intellectual one, but the intellectual function which is disturbed in the congenital reading disability cases is of a higher level than the function which is disturbed in the cases of pure word-blindness."

From this point Schilder went on to examine the probable nature of the essential defect in cases of developmental dyslexia. His observations will be given and discussed later.

Obviously the question of whether the optic perception of verbal symbols is deranged in dyslexics, and if so in what manner, goes right to the heart of the problem.

The early researches of Lucy Fildes (1921) into the fundamental nature of dyslexia are an important contribution. "Word-blindness" was, for her, but one aspect of a more general—yet still specific—defect in either the visual or the auditory regions of the brain, or both. The dyslexic's failure to associate, as well as retain, sounds and forms, lies to some extent in this primary defect, so that forms or sounds fail to gain meaning. Whether there is also a failure in primary retention (and so in the formation of memory-images) could not be determined.

The evidence behind Fildes' conclusions is interesting and important. Her results are unfortunately impaired by the fact that 25 out of her 26 cases were children of low intelligence (I.Q. 50 to 82). Nevertheless she found no close relationship between the intellectual level and the power of reading. Analysis of her patients' performances showed that the inability to read depended upon a specific rather than a general defect. Tests for visual discrimination and for retention of nonsense-forms revealed an impairment among dyslexics far beyond the normal, though there was no lack of speed in perception, nor any failure to recognise the various forms. Fildes concluded that slowness in visual perception is not an important factor in reading difficulties. Non-readers as a class do not find it easy to distinguish between visual impressions which closely resemble each other, although they can readily appreciate and retain differences of greater degree. The failure is due partly to an inability to retain the visual impressions, and partly to slowness of association-processes which hinder the finding of the appropriate name.

Fildes also found that her non-readers as a group displayed a reduction of auditory power, less severe, however, than in the realm of visual material. Incidentally, this is the first point in the history of the dyslexia problem where auditory factors have been raised for discussion.

When tested with random artificial associations between names and Greek letters, dyslexics found this task even harder . . . allegedly because the symbols were so very like each other. This finding supported the conclusion that had already been drawn, namely that it is difficult to forge linkages between names and forms *unless these latter are distinctive in appearance*. This point should be borne in mind when the question is discussed whether the Shavian phonetic alphabet should be adopted widely by teachers or even the augmented Roman alphabet.

Non-readers in Fildes' series made associations between meaningless words and meaningful forms as readily as readers, but their difficulties increased as both forms and sounds grew less distinctive. "Forms and sounds must be readily distinguishable, and both must be meaningful. The essential defect in dyslexia seems to be a failure of forms or sounds to achieve meaning."

Fildes' work leads in a logical fashion to a pictorial "test" for dyslexia, as devised by Maruyama, an electron aviation expert working in Scandinavia. Here non-verbal symbols, differing only in their spatial orientation, are exposed and then matched from a duplicate set (see Fig. 34). Following that, the child is instructed to match the individual cards after the lapse of a short period of time, the model being removed

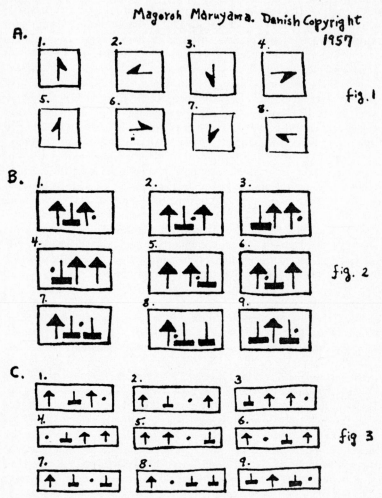

Fig. 34 Maruyama's test using non-verbal symbols.

from sight. In my experience with this test, dyslexics score high marks.

Vernon too (1957) in studying backwardness in reading, could not find in her cases evidence of any general disorder of the visual perception of shapes. There may have been some deficiency in the accurate discrimination of detail and also of spatial orientation, related possibly to a general lack of maturation in analysis and in visual memory. She believed, however, that these defects were likely to be the result (and not the cause) of the reading disability. Of course Vernon was

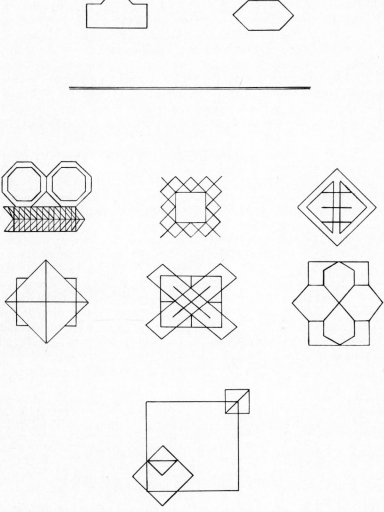

Fig. 35 The Gottschaldt figure test.

studying a widely ranged series of cases where reading skill was slow or retarded, and she explicitly objected to the conception of a specific dyslexia as well as to that term. Her conclusions as to the role of visual perception are important none the less, for her series almost certainly included a number of cases which a neurologist would regard as developmental dyslexics.

In some ways, the results of the various special tests of high visuo-psychic functions in dyslexics, have been contradictory. The accomplishment of the Bender Visual Motor Gestalt test has been noted as inferior when performed by dyslexics (Galifret-Gonjon, 1952). Goins (1958) claimed that there was a correlation between poor reading and defective visual form perception and insecure directional orientation. Lachmann (1960) also found that some dyslexics performed the Bender Visual Motor Gestalt test poorly. Negative findings emerged, however, from the work of Bachmann (1927), Ombredane (1937) and Malmquist (1958). Benton was probably quite correct when he shrewdly pointed out that when visuo-psychic defects were demonstrable in dyslexics it is only so in the case of the younger subjects. He concluded therefrom, that deficiency in visual form perception is *not* an important correlate of developmental dyslexia.

Yet another method of exploring higher visual discrimination which has been applied to retarded readers, is the "embedded figures test". This derives from the Gottschaldt test, as described by Thurstone. A series of simple geometric figures are presented, together with a number of very complex designs (see Fig. 35): the testee is required to detect which of the simple figures lies concealed or incorporated within the complex design. The problem is therefore one of holding or isolating simple figures in elaborate configurations, a task which has been known to be difficult for patients with parieto-occipital lesions. Tjossem *et al.* applied this manœuvre to a series of 16 slow readers and 16 able readers, and the scores were 10·7 and 13·1 respectively. It was concluded that this embedded figure test discriminates between able and slow readers at the age-range 7 to 9 years.

Chapter VIII
Cerebral dominance

That a proportion of dyslexic children were not entirely right-handed subjects was realised early in the history of "congenital word-blindness". With the passage of time increasing importance became attached to this aspect of the problem, and it appeared more and more common to find that dyslexic children were often not endowed with firm and determinate left cerebral dominance. The occurrence of reversals in writing and reading still further directed attention to this problem and a powerful impetus was afforded by the observations of Orton.

Some authors have noted the high incidence of frank left-handedness. Thus, sinistrality was observed in 75% of the cases recorded by Roudinesco, Trelat and Trelat; and in 29% of Dearborn's series. Wall (1945, 1946) also found that 29% of his dyslexics were left-handers as opposed to 14% in a control series. Of Kågen's cases, 15% were left-handed, as compared with 4% among controls. Findings such as these at once throw doubt upon the propriety of the suggestion put forward in 1906 by Clairborne, that dyslexic children should actually be taught to become left-handed. Many other writers, however, could not satisfy themselves as to an increased incidence of left-handedness among the community of poor readers (Monroe, Eames, Gates, Gates and Bond, Witty and Kopel, Bennet, Jackson, Hallgren). Others attached less importance to the role of left-handedness than to left-eyedness, a feature which was found in 27% of Skydsgaard's series (as opposed to 21% in his controls); 40% in Kågen's series (32% in controls); and 100% in Macmeeken's 383 patients. Of the last-named group only 4 were left-handed. Monroe, Dearborn and Crosland also found a higher incidence of left-eyed subjects among poor readers.

Mixed laterality was then imagined to be a factor of special importance in dyslexics who might, for example, prove to be left-eyed, right-handed and left-footed. Any such combination might occur. Thus Orton found mixed eye-hand dominance in 69 out of his 102 cases. Monroe, Dearborn, Eames and Skydsgaard also found a greater proportion of poor readers displaying mixed dominance. But these observations were not confirmed by Gates and Bond, Bennet, Wolfe, Hildreth, Kågen or Hallgren, the last-named commenting upon the inadequacies of most accepted tests of eyedness.

Other writers again have regarded many dyslexics as being "ambidextrous". But nowadays the notion of ambidexterity is realised as being far more complex than hitherto. Eisenson would prefer to speak of a person as being, not ambidextrous, but rather as "ambi-non-dextrous". Many use the term "ambilevity" rather than "ambidexterity".

In any case the inference is that there exists in such individuals no clear-cut dominance of one hemisphere over another. In this respect inadequate cerebral dominance, and mixed laterality, may be considered together, both representing a failure to achieve strong left cerebral suzerainty. This may indeed prove to be a factor of far greater significance in the ætiology of dyslexia than sinistrality itself, whether latent or overt. Thus out of Harris's series of dyslexics (1957), 40% showed mixed dominance (18% in controls) and 25% mixed handedness (8·2% in controls). Of the Chesni cases, 37% showed imperfect laterality. As N. Granjon-Galifret and J. Aguriaguerra put it (1951), "dyslexics are not more often left-handed than normals, but they are more often badly lateralised".

Orton believed that during the normal processes of early visual education, storage of memory-images of letters and words takes place in both hemispheres, and that with the first efforts at learning to read, external visual stimuli irradiate equally into the associative cortices of both hemispheres, and are there represented in both dextrad and sinistrad fashion. The process of learning to read entails the elision from the focus of attention of the confusing memory-images of the non-dominant hemisphere which are in reversed form-order, as well as the selection of those which are in correct orientation and sequence. In cases of reading-disability there has been an incomplete elision of the memory-patterns in the non-dominant hemisphere.

Although this materialistic and over simple hypothesis might not find favour in contemporary thinking, the underlying notion of imperfect cerebral dominance is quite acceptable today as a factor of importance.

An unusual "test" for handedness has been suggested by F. Friedman (1952), who noted the position of the hair-whorl. He estimated the percentage for a right whorl in a normal community to be 21%, and for a left whorl 70%. Applying this sign to a series of retarded readers, T. D. Tjossem, T. J. Hansen and H. S. Ripley (1962) found a right whorl in 54% and a left whorl in 21%. These differences were regarded as significant, and the figures, it was suggested, pointed to a greater than normal tendency to congenital left laterality, despite the fact that the majority of the children were right-handed.

Especially interesting is the Jasper-Raney-Phi test which, by comparing the illusory movement of objects within the two homonymous fields, claims to gauge occipital lobe dominance. Using this test, McFie, and later Ettlinger and Jackson, found that dyslexics display no clear-cut directional preponderance. This suggests a lack of one-sided occipital dominance which may well be the evidence of non-maturation. This state, often spoken of as "cerebral ambilaterality", is believed by some to be associated with an unstable cerebral organisation, one which is particulary sensitive to the effects of stress.

That both cerebral ambilaterality and dyslexia are to be equated with immaturity of cerebral development, is the view most widely held today among neurologists. W. Gooddy and M. Reinhold (1961), who have entertained the same notions of maturational lag, have expressed them in somewhat different terms. They stressed the hypothesis that in normal circumstances asymmetry of the functions of the two cerebral hemispheres is established as a child develops, and that this asymmetry of function is closely related to the performance of reading and writing. Children with developmental dyslexia, however, fail to establish asymmetry of function in the cerebral hemispheres.

Why only a proportion of ill-lateralised children should be dyslexic, is not easy to understand. Some psychologists, especially a decade or two ago, found the conception of sinistrality, as well as of mixed or inadequate dominance, difficult to admit. A. I. Gates and G. L. Bond (1936) objected that eye and hand dominance have little to do with reading-difficulties. Somewhat similar views were put forward by Woody and Phillips (1934); Wolfe (1941); Gates and Bond (1936); Kirk, Teegarden, Witty and Kopel (1936), and others. Vernon (1957) could not understand how incomplete lateralisation and general lack of maturation could explain an inability to learn to read. Not being able to comprehend, she was reluctant to accept the evidence. Theories which attributed reading-disability to some general lack of maturation were, to her, unsatisfactory, in that they gave no explanation as to why reading alone should be affected, and not other cognitive activities. Vernon would have expected some general retardation, or at least slow development of all language-faculties, were the defect due to lack of maturation. She went on to admit, however, that lack of maturation might be a predisposing factor, and that some other factor would be necessary in order to precipitate the disability. Furthermore, she conceded that there might exist a class of individuals who are generally lacking in maturation, who exhibit no well-established laterality, and who show disorders of speech and motility, temperamental instability and reading-disability. Such a condition may be hereditary. Vernon herself gave details of two such cases, and went on to say, "clearly such cases form a small minority of all the cases of reading-disability".

This isolation of an immaturity syndrome is, of course, very reminiscent of what R. S. Eustis had described in 1947. Out of a pedigree comprising 33 descendants, 14 displayed one or more features of a "syndrome" comprising speech delay or defect; left-handedness or ambidexterity; clumsiness; and also specific reading-disability. Eustis looked upon this syndrome as representing a rather specialised delay in development, and he spoke of a slow tempo of neuro-muscular maturation, probably indicative of a slow myelination of motor and association nerve tracts.

Undoubtedly, however, a fair number of dyslexics are unequivocal dextrals with no family history of left-handedness or ambidexterity. In the absence of any greater correlation it is therefore tempting to invoke a hypothesis which would seek to explain the occurrence of dyslexia upon an underlying delayed, or incomplete, lateralisation of cerebral function. Zangwill (1962) has wondered whether there might be two sorts of developmental dyslexia, namely a type occurring in poorly lateralised individuals, as contrasted with a type presenting in individuals who are lateralised fully. He had indeed been struck by the frequent association of retarded speech development, defects of spatial perception, motor clumsiness and related indications of defective maturation in cases of dyslexia presenting in ill-lateralised (and some left-handed) children. On the other hand, Zangwill was impressed by the comparative "purity" of the dyslexia when it presents itself in fully right-handed children, and he suggested that a specific genetical factor might plausibly be assumed in this particular group.

The relationship between types of cerebral dominance and the occurrence of dyslexia is, however, complicated by two factors which have but incompletely been clarified in the literature. In the first place the question of handedness is a much more complex problem than is generally understood, and handedness cannot be definitely established upon the basis of any single one clinical "test". A veritable battery of tests is needed to determine the factor of handedness, and this may often turn out to be a relative matter. That is to say a child may be only "relatively" right-handed or left-handed, as judged by the formula of manual skills and postures. The second point is the fact that in correlating handedness with dyslexia it has often been only too obvious that the author was using a material made up of diverse types of poor reading ability, not all of which were true cases of developmental dyslexia.

Zangwill has been struck by the fact that only some ill-lateralised children have reading-problems. He put forward three possible explanations which could be offered. The first possible idea is that poorly developed laterality and reading-defect could both be due to the effects of an acutal cerebral lesion. A second hypothesis is that the reading difficulty and the lack of cerebral asymmetry could both be taken as evidence of a constitutional maturational lag. The third possibility— and this is the one which Zangwill seems cautiously to favour—is that the children who lack firm lateral preferences are particularly vulnerable to the effects of stress—though how this last condition conduces to dyslexia was not pursued.

Chapter IX
Minor neurological signs

Despite what has been asserted, cases of "specific" or developmental dyslexia are not always entirely "pure" in the sense that the disability may not exist in complete isolation. This statement in no way detracts from the neurological conception of developmental dyslexia as a specific constitutional genetically determined defect lying within the middle zone of a spectrum of non-specific reading disorders. The occasional "impurity" of the syndrome is shown by the elucidation at times, on appropriate testing, of various minor deficits, or "soft" neurological signs, as they have been called in the U.S.A. Some of these are virtually "minimal" and may elude superficial examination, coming to light only after more searching techniques. Many of these little signs are related to an incomplete maturation of the nervous system, and they are more likely to be found among the younger age-groups, being rarer in dyslexics who have attained adolescence. This is well shown by the battery of tests used by Mrs. de Hirsch for the prediction of dyslexics at the $5\frac{1}{2}$–$6\frac{1}{2}$ year level.

The principal deficits which may be brought to light on appropriate testing by what Rabinovitch called the "expanded" neurological examination, include the following: (1) disorders of spatial thought; (2) impaired temporal notions; (3) inadequate, inconsistent, or mixed cerebral dominance; (4) defects of speech or of language, other than dyslexia; (5) disorders of motility; and (6) poor figure-background discrimination. The last two are especially important in very young subjects.

Disorders of spatial thought and spatial manipulation are important even though they may be demonstrable only in the minority of cases.

The statement made by Gooddy and Reinhold (1961) that there is invariably a right-left disorientation of some degree goes perhaps too far. The spatial disabilities recall those met with in adult patients with parietal lobe lesions, differing however in that they are manifesting themselves at an earlier age, and that they are less flamboyant and less outstanding. As in parietal disease they are highly diverse in their appearances. German writers have referred to a *Labilität der Raumlage* (instability of spatial notions) in this setting.

Spatial disabilities may be clearly displayed in the spontaneous drawings executed by dyslexics. Often there is a conspicuous lack of perspective in, say, pictures of a house. Or there may be a dimensional confusion so that elevation and plan are jumbled up in an odd manner. Even greater spatial defects may at times be shown when the dyslexic tries to model with plasticine and to construct simple three-dimensional figures or shapes. The dyslexic child often mixes up the extra-corporeal spatial directions such as up and down, and more often still, left and right. Prepositions such as "on", "under", "below", "behind", "beyond" may prove incomprehensible or may be confused. In attempting to write or to make arithmetical calculations, the child may set down the words and figures upon the paper in an irregular and even haphazard fashion. Figures and words are not placed under each other in correct alignment: the left-hand margins are too narrow or too wide, and often they descend obliquely.

Again, as in the case of acquired parietal disease in the adult, spatial disorders may be combined with other considerations—related perhaps to topography, corporeal awareness, constructional tasks, or motor performance. Thus the dyslexic child may be quite unable to draw a plan or chart of a familiar room or locality. He may also be unable to read a map or street-plan; to set the hands of a clock to command; to direct strangers in the street to familiar places; or to "navigate" the parent who is driving a car.

Spatial manipulations which entail an accurate notion of corporeal awareness (body-image) may be found to be faulty in such tasks as dressing. Especially difficult is the manœuvre of fastening shoe-laces and of knotting a bow tie. More obvious is the right and left confusion already alluded to, and most interesting of all, an inability to name or to indicate the individual fingers. Of greater complexity are the tasks which entail the "crossing of the mid-line of the body", and the dyslexic child may find it difficult to do manipulations with the right hand to its left, and with the left hand to its right.

A variant of spatial disorientation is the phenomenon of confusion between right and left in ordinary semi-automatic activities. Though this is not wholly unknown in normal subjects it is certainly more often encountered in those who are backward in reading. The confusion in lateral dimensions may pass unnoticed until special circumstances bring it into the open. Thus when the poor reader is called up into the Armed Forces he may mix up his right and his left in the barrack square to a degree which transcends the usual awkwardness of a recruit. In the Navy the new-entry may muddle up port and starboard. According to Hermann an officer in the Danish army was interested to observe that recruits who had been selected for special coaching because of illiteracy were also those who had been notorious for their right–left confusion at squad drill. Hermann also referred to the case of a taxi-driver in Copenhagen who was so word-blind that he could not cope with his necessary book-work, and who was also hopelessly inept at distinguishing right from left. To surmount this latter defect he was in the habit of putting a black mark on the right thumbnail when directed by a passenger in an unfamiliar suburb. To anticipate such a contingency, he always carried a piece of black chalk in his pocket. When necessary he would surreptitiously blacken his right thumbnail before attending to instructions to turn this way or that.

More banal disorders entailing both motility and spatial notions are seen in those dyslexics who are poor at ball-games; who cannot catch a ball in flight; or who take an unconscionable time to learn to ride a bicycle or a scooter. Constructional tasks which embrace spatial concepts, include the assembling of jig-saw puzzles, a game which may not be easy for some of these dyslexics. This difficulty is readily assessed by the test of Kohs' blocks, where some dyslexics fare badly.

A simple "reversible figures test" has been used to gauge the ability of a patient to reproduce simple figures after a brief delay, and to note the frequency of errors of a reversal type. A card containing an assymmetrical design is exposed for three seconds and then removed: the patient, after an interval of another three seconds, is required to draw the design on paper. A series of such cards is used and the number of reversals is noted. Children who are poor readers appear to score badly with this test, indicating a difficulty with the perceptual stabilisation of figures. Tjossem *et al.* found that reversals and rotations were common with this test up to the age of $8\frac{1}{2}$ years in slow readers, the mean rotational score being 3·4. Over the age of $8\frac{1}{2}$, however, this kind of defect was less common, the mean rotational score being now only 0·4. The tendency to reversals and rotations of symbols was more pronounced within the population of slow readers, the tendency diminishing, however, with age.

Closely bound up with disorders of spatial thought in dyslexics, are the evidences of inadequate temporal notions. Ideas of "sequence" are of particular importance in that they combine conceptions which are of both a spatial and temporal nature. Sequential disorders are of extreme importance in dyslexics for they may point to the fundamental nature of the underlying defect. Some dyslexics show an imperfect sense of rhythm. There are some who cannot recite in correct serial order the days of the week or months of the year, and who confuse the time-incidence of important occasions in history. This failure to enumerate correctly the calendar months was specially noted by Engler, and by Laubenthal. L. Bender also stressed these temporal defects. In her series of dyslexic children she found some who muddled past, present and future, and who could not understand the various tenses of the verbs. Terms such as "now", "then", tomorrow", "yesterday" had but little meaning for them. To some of her children the phrase "the first day of the week" meant very little, for they saw no more reason for starting on the left-hand side of the calendar with a Sunday, than on the right with a Saturday. Learning to read the time was a delayed accomplishment in some of the dyslexics, and one child asked why it was that the long hand of the clock was for the minutes and the short hand for the hours, when hours were so much longer than minutes. Memory of past events were not well organised and one child could not indicate in correct sequence the outstanding events which had happened to her.

In later life the dyslexic may experience considerable difficulty in learning Morse signalling. Indeed, it was this particular disability which brought a problem Royal Naval cadet to my notice during the war (Critchley, 1942).

Certain authors, and especially those who have associated developmental dyslexia with a global retardation in the acquisition of language, have drawn attention to the co-existence of disorders of speech in dyslexic children. Some have emphasised a comparatively late age at which the child uttered its first word, or strung together words in logical fashion to form phrases or sentences. An immature or dyslexic disorder of speaking has often been observed though usually it proves to be merely a transient phenomenon. Thus disorders of articulation or of the development of articulate speech have been reported in 30% of the cases observed by B. Kågen (1943); 41% of the boys and 32% of the girls in the dyslexics studied by B. Hallgren (1952); in certain of Ingram's cases (1959); and in 16 out of the 23 dyslexics described by F. H. Hibbert (1961). Besides late development of speech, and imperfections in articulation, there may also be demonstrable at times an immaturity of the faculty of language as opposed to speech. Thus inadequacies or immaturity in syntax and in vocabulary may at times be discerned. For example, the child may emit what might be called reversals of concepts, e.g. black for white, nice for nasty. Direction is frequently muddled but it is often difficult to decide whether it is a spatial or a linguistic defect. R. E. Saunders has also referred to reversals of time-sequences, whereby the dyslexic child may say first for last, now for later, seldom for often. One child within his series said "the day after yesterday . . . I mean the day before tomorrow": when what he really meant was the day after tomorrow (1962). However, these disorders of language and of diction are far from being invariable, and they are best regarded as being epiphenomena.

Faust has drawn attention to two curious defects which he has noticed in association with developmental dyslexia, and which suggest a highest level visual dysgnosia. In the first place there was an odd inability on the part of the dyslexic child to interpret the meaning of people's facial expressions, especially when in pictorial form. Secondly, he observed a veritable simultanagnosia, that is, an inability to grasp the meaning of a picture as a whole. In my experience of dyslexics, interpretation of both facial expressions and of pictures has been strikingly accurate and even shrewd. Yet another complicated visual defect in dyslexics—which has already been mentioned—is the difficulty in distinguishing colours and also in naming them correctly. This has been specifically reported by Warburg.

Chief among the motility-disorders which can at times be discerned in dyslexic children is a general *gaucherie* or awkwardness. The gait may be shambling. The child may run in an ungainly fashion, and frequently tumble. Manual dexterity may be so poor as to raise the suspicion of a "congenital" type of motor dyspraxia. Because of muscular inco-ordination the dyslexic child may find it hard to bounce a ball, to tie and untie knots, or to fasten and unfasten buttons. These shortcomings were particularly stressed by Rabinovitch and his colleagues (1954) who wrote, "observation of gait, and the performance of motor acts such as dressing, opening and closing doors, and the handling of psychological test-materials, led to the definite impression of a non-specific awkwardness and clumsiness in motor function".

L. Bender has repeatedly drawn attention to the persistence of tonic neck reflex dominance, a phenomenon which normally disappears at the age of $6\frac{1}{2}$ to $7\frac{1}{2}$ years.

When the Bender Gestalt battery of tests is put to dyslexic children, several complicated motor-spatio-constructional defects may be uncovered. (1) The figures often tend to be primitive, "fluid" and full of movement of the vertical, whirling type; (2) squared figures become rounded, dots are replaced by loops, diamonds tend to be squared and oblique lines become vertical or even horizontal; (3) there is some disorientation of the background, usually by rotation of mobile figures, or by "verticalisation"; (4) open figures are apt to be closed; and (5) there is a tendency for the child to convert figures, especially those that are verticalised and closed, into a man by drawing a face within the enclosure.

F. M. Lachmann (1960) studying dyslexics by way of the Bender Gestalt test found a five-fold type of distortion, viz. angulation, rotation, primitivation, separation and slant. The presence of these distortions, especially in the younger age-groups readily distinguishes children with reading-disabilities from normal subjects. But emotionally disturbed normal readers also often showed these same distortions. Other authors had previously noted some of these types of distortion (e.g. rotation by Fabian, 1945; angulation by Silver, 1953; and primitivation by de Hirsch, 1954).

It has already been stated that some dyslexics—though certainly not all—may fare badly at arithmetic. Apart from a slowness in identifying numerical symbols, there may be an incapacity to grasp ideas of number and of relative size. The principles underlying addition, subtraction, multiplication and division may never be mastered, constituting a true developmental dyscalculia. Again, there are two other interesting and not unrelated disabilities which have already been referred to, namely a disorientation in lateral dimension, and a finger-agnosia. Immediately one is reminded of a Gerstmann's syndrome, with its four cardinal components of dysgraphia, dyscalculia, right-left disorientation and finger-agnosia, following a lesion of the dominant parietal lobe. Could dyslexia therefore be a manifestation of an inherent Gerstmann's syndrome, as was originally suggested by Hermann and Norrie?

Both dyslexia and Gerstmann's syndrome have been ascribed by some to a common factor of directional dysfunction, the result of a failure of lateral orientation with reference to corporeal awareness, and the organisation of self within extra-personal space. However important, this point can scarcely be fundamental, for a Gerstmann syndrome is certainly not an integral part of dyslexia. Right-left confusion is common; finger-agnosia much less so; while dyscalculia may be wholly absent. Both Benton (1958, 1959, 1962) and A. J. Harris (1957) have, on the contrary, found that the incidence of right-left disorientation is only slightly higher in dyslexics than in normal readers.

A. C. Benton and J. D. Kemble (1960) were sceptical, believing that dyslexics show only a mild tendency towards a malperformance of higher order right-left orientation-exercises. This they interpret as a reflection of a relative impairment in symbolisation and conceptualisation. Benton is, of course, critical of the whole notion of Gerstmann's syndrome as an entity.

J. Money has stressed the confusion between visual and body images which seems to underlie the difficulties of directional orientation in dyslexics. Their problem is not merely a simple one of right-left confusion, nor yet one of difficulty with perception of form in two dimensions. "It is truly a three-dimensional *space-movement* perception problem, involving the relationship of the visual image to the body image in ahead and behind, toward and away-from, left and right, and facing upward or downward."

In concluding an account of the minor neurological signs which may at times be demonstrated in dyslexics, reference may be made to the occurrence of high-level sensory disturbances, as claimed by Rabinovitch *et al.* These authors found delay in the appreciation of double face-hand tactile stimuli; inaccurate localisation of touch; and impaired two-point discrimination.

In recapitulating the diverse neurological disorders which may be uncovered after close and particular scrutiny, it must be stressed that these findings are by no means integral. Many a dyslexic—perhaps even the majority of cases—show no such disabilities, despite the most alerted and scrupulous testing-procedures. Perhaps they should be regarded as important epiphenomena—significant when they occur, but not essential in any consideration as to pathogenesis or ætiology. When these neurological manifestations are found, there seems to be an inverse correlation with the age of the patients. In other words, the younger the subject the more likely it is that neurological signs will be found, while with older dyslexics the greater the likelihood of a negative clinical examination.

Some authors, it is true, have tried to isolate certain neurological groupings and to relate them in a causal fashion with the occurrence of dyslexia. We have already referred to the Hermann-Norrie notion of a developmental Gerstmann syndrome. Silver and Hagin (1960) were able to demonstrate in 92% of their cases, a syndrome comprising: (1) Visuo-motor immaturity; (2) specific difficulty in spatial orientation (angulation difficulties; confusion in figure-background perception); (3) inability to grasp the temporal relationships of sounds; and (4) body-image distortion, with "tonus and postural problems".

The neurological conspectus of developmental dyslexia includes the evidence of electro-encephalography. Its role is admittedly minor in character. Mild dysrhythmias are often found, suggestive of cortical immaturity, and these may be most evident in the parieto-occipital areas bilaterally.

Neuro-psychological findings in dyslexics necessarily differ in many respects according to the age of the subject. As already mentioned, the neurological anomalies are likely to be more conspicuous in dyslexics of the younger age-group. In adult dyslexics the diagnosis is relatively easier provided one can estimate and allow for possible psychiatric overlays. The problem is more difficult in very young children, where cases of true specific dyslexia have to be identified and distinguished from children who are backward in learning to read for other reasons, such as general intellectual retardation. The series of tests described by de Hirsch is therefore a useful guide to diagnosis. At the early age of 5½ years the putative dyslexics often show themselves to be fidgety children (this feature has been independently noted by M. Creak). Their movements are jerky and clumsy. Isolated skilled movements may be replaced by global motor responses. Their spontaneous drawings may be revealing.

As a well-documented study of a very young dyslexic we may quote the case of "Dick" reported by Jansky (1958).

Dick was of superior intelligence and unusual charm. Besides his presenting problem in learning to read, he was mildly inco-ordinate, as evidenced by his drawings. He could not recall the names of colours. Time, as a framework, had but little meaning for him; he had no verbal concepts of "yesterday" or "tomorrow". References to the future were extremely vague. He seemed to lack a clear feeling of separation from surrounding space. Thus, unlike most of the children attending the Clinic, he preferred to work in the very smallest rooms, saying, "I feel lost in the playroom—this one is not so loose". Out of doors he was liable to get lost. As to the orientation of printed symbols, it was all the same to him whether the words went from left to right, or the other way. For him the beginning of a word could just as well have been the end. When he tried to read aloud he found it hard to adhere to the line, and on reaching a difficult word he was apt to slip into the line above or the line below. In the case of verbal symbols the visual complex was, for him, all-important. Thus while he might manage to read a word printed in black letters on a yellow card, the same word on a white card would be impossible. Throughout the examination Dick showed himself unable to abstract or to generalise, being everlastingly bogged down in his concrete way of thinking.

The detailed study of an adult dyslexic made by Pflugfelder makes an interesting comparison, for additional points could be determined.

The patient proved to be a strong eidetic. This faculty obviously entails certain advantages, such as an enhanced visual imagery and recall. But there may also be drawbacks. Although eidetics can readily conceive and retain within the optic sphere an object as a whole, the deliberate breaking-down of the whole into its constituent parts is more difficult for them, precisely because the whole is conceived with abnormal ease. What is an advantage when it comes to visualising and memorising geometric forms, acts as a handicap in reading and writing. This patient's behaviour in a visual context was always concrete and non-analytic, as shown by tests with optical illusions and ambiguous figures which provoked none of the usual reaction of hesitancy and indecision.

Pflugfelder's patient is all the more interesting in that the strong eidetic imagery of his dyslexic patient seems to run counter to what other writers upon dyslexia have imagined to occur. In the Johns Hopkins symposium upon Dyslexia (1961) there were references to the notion that the dyslexic was a subject who has difficulty not only in establishing the necessary lexical concepts, visual and auditory, and in relating the visual and phonic images, but is also in some way a non-visile cognitional type. As Money said, he is perhaps a person weak in visual imagery and visual memory of all types, the opposite of the person with eidetic imagery and photographic memory.

Chapter X
Genetic properties

We owe to genetics the most cogent single argument in support of the conception of a constitutional specific type of dyslexia identifiable among the miscellany of cases of poor readers. Although as long ago as 1905 it was observed that congenital word-blindness might involve more than one member of a family, this aspect attracted little notice at first. The pioneer here was C. J. Thomas who found six patients within two generations of a single family. In the same year F. Herbert Fisher recorded congenital word-blindness in an uncle and a nephew. The following year S. Stephenson went so far as to postulate a recessive mode of inheritance on the basis of six cases cropping up in three generations. Hinshelwood and also McCready observed a familial occurrence. Plate (1910) found poor readers among three generations. (Later the same phenomenon was to be recorded by Marshall and Ferguson (1939) and by H. Rønne (1936).) In 1911 Warburg of Cologne ventured the opinion that dyslexia was often transmitted by the unaffected mother. He also stressed the important point that the information supplied by a parent is not always wholly reliable, for there is a tendency to "play down" the familial incidence. Illing (1929) who found hereditary factors in seven out of eleven cases, discovered that in three of his patients both parents were poor readers. Laubenthal of Bonn published a complicated pedigree in which dyslexia was associated with many examples of mental defect, criminal propensity, and psychopathy. Writing in 1936 he asserted that in severe cases of word-blindness it was justifiable to carry out sterilisation.

Scandinavian researchers have since afforded valuable evidence as to the importance of genetic factors in dyslexia. Norrie (1939) found familial tendencies in "practically all" of her cases. Kågen (1943) mentioned 30%, and Ramer (1947) 50 to 60%. Skydsgaard (1942) published a number of pedigrees which obviously revealed a genetical factor, though of uncertain nature. Most important has been the monograph of B. Hallgren (1950) based upon 276 cases, all but six being personally observed. In his experience 88% of all cases had reading problems in one or more other members of the family. The cases were made up of children attending the Stockholm Child Guidance Clinic, and children from either a Folkskola or a Larsverk, i.e. elementary or secondary schools; Hallgren divided his material into four groups in the following manner: *Group 1*. Families with "secondary cases" (i.e. proband's sibs and *both* parents affected with specific dyslexia) (3 probands and 8 secondary cases); *Group 2*. Families with seconda cases and *one* parent affected (94 probands and 147 secondary cases);

Group 3. Families with both parents unaffected and cases of specific dyslexia among the proband's sibs, sibs of their parents, or grandparents of the probands (7 probands and 5 secondary cases); and *Group 4.* Solitary cases (12). The author concluded that developmental dyslexia follows a monohybrid autosomal dominant mode of inheritance. Furthermore Hallgren, and also Norrie, made studies upon twins with dyslexia. The total number of pairs investigated was 45, of which 12 were monozygotic and 33 dizygotic. There was a 100% concordance among the former group, as opposed to 33% among the latter. Other instances of dyslexia among identical twins have been described by Brander (1935), Ley and Tordeur (1936), Jenkins, Brown and Elmendorf (1937), and by Schiller (1937).

Vernon adopted a rather critical attitude towards the genetic factor in cases of retarded reading, and in her scepticism of the existence of a specific form of dyslexia, she found it difficult to accept Hallgren's conclusion that specific reading disability is in most cases a single and isolated congenital disability. She required further corroborative evidence from other studies, despite the minute care and skill with which Hallgren assembled and analysed his material. Vernon thought it more plausible to assert that there is a congenital disposition in certain cases towards the occurrence of certain related defects: reading disability; speech-defects or infantile speech; motor incoordination; left-handedness or ambidexterity. But, seven years before, Hallgren had expressly examined and unequivocally stated that his present study lent no support to the hypothesis that specific dyslexia, mental deficiency, nervous disorders, left-handedness and speech defects were different phenotypical manifestations of the same hereditary taint.

It has almost always been observed that developmental dyslexia affects males more often than females, though Jastak could find no sex difference in his series. The estimate varies from one author to another.

The table on page 65 illustrates the reported sex-incidence as determined by a number of authors.

We can therefore assume that about 4 males to 1 female may be accepted as a reasonable figure.

Again, Vernon is out of concord on the question of sex-incidence. She believed that the claimed preponderance of boys was due to her allegation that non-readers among boys create more trouble at school than do non-readers among girls; or at least they bring their disability more forcibly to the teacher's notice, while girls suffer in silence. Perhaps too, Vernon surmised, parents take a more serious view of inability to read in a boy than in a girl. The explanation, however, which Vernon deemed most likely was that boys with reading disability had superadded emotional disorders, these being frequently aggressive

TABLE III

Author	Year	Percentage of Males	Total number in series
Bachmann . .	1927	70	80
Illing . . .	1929	80	12
Anderson & Kelley.	1931	84	100
Monroe . . .	1932	84	50
Brander . . .	1935	100	12
Blanchard . .	1936	86	73
Witty & Kopel .	1936	66	100
Creak . . .	1936	76	50
Bennet . . .	1938	72	50
Skydsgaard . .	1942	80	26
Orton . . .	1943	82	102
Eames . . .	1944	80	100
Wallin . . .	1949	82	120
Norman . .	1950	76·8	694
Hallgren . .	1950	76	116

by nature. Boys are referred to clinics because these latter disorders have brought them to the notice of teachers and parents rather than the disability itself.

These observations—and particularly the last—would not tally with the experience of neurological consultants to whom children with dyslexia are brought by worried parents entirely on account of their paradoxical inability to learn to read. Among such children the boys unquestionably outnumber the girls.

To date no connection has yet been found between dyslexia and chromosomal aberrations, as based upon recent techniques of intracellular chromosome counting.

The question may be discussed whether the position of the dyslexic child within the birth series is important in this connection. Warburg, it will be recalled, invoked the notion of maternal *Produktionserschöpfung* and he had the idea that dyslexia was most likely to occur in the youngest member of a large family. His conclusions were based upon the small series of 21 families. Twenty years later Anderson and Kelley, dealing with a group of 100 cases of reading disability, found a significantly smaller number of solitary children, or of eldest children, affected with dyslexia. They believed that paternal solicitude was more likely to be operative in the case of an only child who was backward in years, or in a first child. Bennet too, in 1938, found a smaller number of eldest children (8 out of 50) affected with dyslexia as compared with a control group of 17 out of 50 where the first-born was not affected. Hallgren (1950) went into the problem of ordinal position much more carefully than previous authors. He found that children with dyslexia are distributed among the different numbers in the birth series. Thus, out of his total case-material 79·5 cases were found in the first half of the sibship and 100·5 among the second half.

With regard to any possible relationship between dyslexia and consanguineous parenthood Hallgren found no supporting evidence.

Reference may be made to the occasional occurrence of an inherent asymbolia for musical notation, which has been described as alternating with cases of dyslexia from one generation to another (Hermann).

Chapter XI
The size of the problem

Here lies a particularly difficult question. The percentage of dyslexics within the community has been overestimated by some writers. Others again have surely underestimated the magnitude of the problem. Among this latter group must surely belong the figures contained in the Ministry of Education's "Health of the Schoolchild in 1960 and 1961". A few extremists even decry the very existence of dyslexia. The explanation for the divergence of opinion lies partly in the difficulties in diagnosis, but more especially, in the personal prejudices of the observer. Possibly the proportion of dyslexics is not the same in different countries. Developmental dyslexics tend to be submerged within the larger population of bad readers, and so their specificity may escape detection. Years ago Nettleship shrewdly asserted that congenital word-blindness was easy to detect in the children of well-educated parents, diagnosis being much more difficult in children who crowd our infant elementary schools.

There is an added problem which crops up when trying to estimate the frequency of dyslexia, namely the effort to disentangle these specific cases out of the general population of educationally retarded individuals. Within the latter category belong the facultative illiterates, which according to Gray, constitute 50% of the world's population, at least another 15% being "nearly illiterate".

We learn too that out of New York's juvenile delinquents in 1955 no fewer than 75% were illiterate (Harrower). The same percentage has been found in France where out of a population of young offenders (12 to 16 years of age) in Paris the proportion of non-readers was said to have been at least 75%. Aside from delinquency Bauer (1959) opined that eight million retarded readers exist in the United States of America at the present time. According to Rabinovitch and his colleagues about 10% of all American children of average intelligence read so badly that their total adjustment is impaired. To what extent these groupings represent a mélange of the educationally inadequate, the intellectually deficient, the emotionally disturbed, the infirm of purpose, and the genuine dyslexics, has never been determined. The same uncertainty is attached to figures from England and Wales, prepared by the Ministry of Education, wherein in 1950 1·4% of all 15-year-old youngsters were found to be illiterate. By "illiteracy" was understood a reading ability of less than 7 years by the standards of 1938, while a reading ability of between 7 and 8 years was regarded as indicating "semi-illiteracy". This latter group amounted to 4·3%. In each case "silent" reading is implied. The 1956 figures from the Ministry of Education estimated that 15% of all adults belong to the class of illiterates and semi-literates.

Reverting to the estimations that have been made by those authors who have dealt specifically with dyslexia, we find that Thomas (1905) guessed that one in every two thousand schoolchildren were congenitally word-blind. By 1909 McCready reckoned that 41 cases had been described within the world's literature, mainly from British and American sources. Subsequent authors put the incidence higher. Thus Wallin (1911) found dyslexia in 0·7% of a series of schoolchildren. Hallgren (1950) judged the incidence in Sweden of specific dyslexia within the normal population, as roughly 10%. Sinclair (1948), Hermann (1959), Rabino-vitch *et al.* (1954) each gauged the occurrence as around 10%. Childs (1959) said 5·5% to 25%, Silver and Hagin (1960), 5% to 25%, and Bender (1957) believed that between 5% and 15% of all schoolchildren were unable to acquire language-skills as rapidly as most youngsters with comparable intellectual ability and schooling. In 1951 there existed in Denmark 151 "special reading classes" where over 2,500 children attended: this figure did not include the pupils at the Hellerup Word-blind Institute.

Neurologists believe that true, specific, developmental dyslexia is a comparatively rare condition, although it must be admitted that there is still no scientific evidence available for the precise incidence to be determined. Here neurologists would entirely agree with Vernon when she asserted that we have no evidence as to the frequency of congenital reading disability among backward readers in general, and that it is unlikely that they constitute more than a small proportion even of severe cases of reading-disability. Doubtless, however, dyslexia is commoner than generally imagined. Cases are constantly being overlooked by teachers, and misinterpreted by educational psychologists. Although Hermann's figure of 10% of dyslexics among Danish schoolchildren tallies exactly with Sinclair's survey of primary schools in Edinburgh, I should have judged this figure as almost certainly too high for England.

At the same time the problem is grave enough and sufficiently important to justify official recognition. Facilities should be made for the early recognition of dyslexics, followed by opportunities for these children to receive individual, sympathetic, and intensive tuition, either in special classes or in special schools, residential or otherwise. An even more satisfactory solution might be in the training of a corps of specialised teachers of dyslexia, who could be sent to schools in sufficient numbers to deal with children who had been screened and later accepted as victims of developmental dyslexia. The problem is one which requires the active participation of neurologists at the diagnostic stage.

Chapter XII
Psychiatric repercussions

Developmental dyslexics and indeed all children with difficulty in learning to read, tend at a quite early age to develop neurotic reactions. Sometimes these are severe and may lead to a striking personality change. Nothing could be more natural. Some of the autobiographical accounts written by adult sufferers have been eloquent and quite moving in the narration of their life-long predicaments.* The dyslexic is apt to find himself an alien in a critical, if not hostile, milieu; mocked, misunderstood, or penalised; cut off from opportunities for advancement. Should the dyslexic child be of high intelligence, his prospects of developing neurotic reactions may be all the greater, as he sees himself lagging behind junior members of his family, and younger companions. As an adolescent, the dyslexic occupies a ridiculous position especially in his contacts with the other sex, being handicapped socially, unable to read menus, programmes, film titles or news items; and incapable of receiving or writing letters. In adult life the dyslexic is bereft of intellectual and cultural advantages; professional careers are barred. He is doomed to a second-class citizenship, for he is blind to the printed instructions, warnings, appeals, exhortations and information which surround him. Rabinovitch et al. who, it will be recalled, emphasised a distinction between primary and secondary types of reading retardation, believed that patients belonging to the secondary group showed more evidences of a "negative" character. But those with a primary reading retardation (who would correspond with our specific developmental dyslexics) have a high motivation to learn to read.

There is probably nothing specific or uniform about the neurotic pattern which may develop. The psychiatric features have been rated as pleomorphic and even at times bizarre. However, the ease with which a dyslexic teenager slips into delinquency demands serious notice. Von Holstein, a Danish High Court Judge, has made a special study of the correlation of word-blindness with criminal propensity.

Fortunately the neurotic reactions of dyslexics—however severe— are usually benign in character, for they readily yield to treatment, once the underlying basis of difficulty in reading is realised and handled sympathetically.

The foregoing opinions as to the neurotic overlay are not universally held, however. Some believe the neurotic picture to be clinically

---

* See, for example, the letter written by Axel Rosendal (quoted by Hermann); the article by "X" in the Brit. J. Ophth., 1936; Skydsgaard's account of the ex-word-blind lawyer; and the description retailed by Hermann, pp. 158–60.

a specific one. L. Bender described the personality of the dyslexic as immature, impulse-ridden and dependent, and that he is often mistakenly regarded as post-encephalitic, retarded or schizophrenic. Scores of the intelligence quotient may differ widely in the same child at different interviews. With the Rorschach test, dyslexics are said to be characterised by reason of their pure colour responses; colour shock, and poor form visualisation; immaturity; disturbances in emotional development; and social adaptation (E. Gann, 1945). McCready (1926–27) claimed that he could recognise a number of patterns of neurotic response in word-blind children, such as (1) a contented, apathetic disregard of the handicap and its results; (2) a mild paranoid reaction towards the teachers, leading to behavioural disorders, truancy and depredations upon school property; (3) a profound sense of inferiority; and (4) emotional blocking, consisting for the most part in a halt in output when anything is demanded as a task or assignment.

The age at which a child normally begins to read with facility is also the age at which—according to Piaget—he turns from an autistic, egocentric individual, to a societal, ethnocentric being. It has been suggested that the very act of successfully learning to read plays an important part in this normal phase of externalisation (J. M. Wepman). The non-reader or dyslexic may continue for an undue length of time at his stage of autism. Perhaps this hypothesis goes some way towards explaining the occasional lapses into delinquency.

Again, there are writers who imply, even if they do not state explicitly, that the neurotic symptoms in poor readers are causal rather than reactionary. Various psychoanalytic hypotheses of reading-disability may be quoted for the record, and for what they are worth. Three supposedly related factors have been inculpated, namely: fear and avoidance of looking; hostility, primarily towards the same-sex parent; and failure to identify with the same-sex parent. R. H. Walters, M. Van Loan and I. Crofts (1961) put these ideas to the test in a series of poor readers. These children performed less well on two perceptual tasks which involved recognition of form. They were slower at opening a compartment to look for a male nude doll than were the average or advanced readers used as controls. In addition they chose their father less often in a simple parent-preference test. On the other hand, fantasy data failed to support the "fear of looking" notion or the hostility hypothesis. A confusion of right and left, and a tendency towards reversals of letters or words has been equated by Jones, Abraham and other analysts, not with lack of spatial co-ordination but with traits of aural eroticism. Some analysts take up an indeterminate or midway attitude and blame a neurotic inadequacy, whereby there exists a tendency to avoid any situation demanding sustained attention at a difficult or boring intellectual task. Learning to read may fall within this category and consequently suffer in a seemingly specific fashion.

Thus Mildred Creak (1936) wrote "in so far as these children (i.e. poor readers) have any sort of emotional difficulty common to the group, it would seem to be an aversion to effort, showing itself in distractability, restlessness and lack of interest in books, and granted some common basis for the initial difficulty in reading, it is easy to see how the habitual evasion of that difficulty will tend to set up faulty associations, and a persistence of these, until the mistakes become a habitual reaction".

H. F. R. Prechtl (1962) already referred to, has also adopted a sort of compromise attitude. He isolated a group of young patients with reading difficulty in whom there are conspicuous choreiform movements. These not only involve the motor act of reading, but they also produce a serious instability of concentration. Prechtl's description does not convince one that this problem has any important application to cases of specific developmental dyslexia.

Even today the all too common tendency is for observers, including some teachers and many child psychiatrists, to fail to realise that the neurotic symptoms which a dyslexic may show, are secondary or reactionary. Only too often the backwardness in reading is deemed either an environmental, or a psychogenic problem, or both, causing a reluctance on the part of the child to persevere with the uphill task of learning his letters. So injustice is done: the specific defect which may well be present is overlooked; and the dyslexic remains misunderstood and untaught.

Incidentally, it is of no little interest to turn to the obverse of the coin, and to note that a correlation has been traced by Lynn (1955), between anxiety in children, and a precocious or supernormal facility in reading.

Dyslexics who are of high intelligence and who are also fortunate enough to retain their emotional stability, are sometimes capable of high achievement in later life. If the specific disability has been recognised for what it is, and if there has been intensive and sympathetic coaching, the patient may lose many of his difficulties with reading, spelling and writing. Furthermore, by resorting to an auditory system of learning, and by fostering such potentialities as memory and quick associations, the dyslexic may still further advance in his schooling, and may even master or circumvent the screening processes which threaten to debar him from a career. According to an autobiographical account, one such dyslexic patient even attained high rank in the Foreign Office. One of Wernicke's patients became a lawyer. Another dyslexic is known to have become a surgeon, who acquired his knowledge from lectures and bedside tuition rather than from books, and whose written work was legible enough to secure a pass. Yet another became an instructor in a military academy (Plate, 1909). It has even been alleged that the famous John Hunter was a dyslexic, but the evidence advanced to support that contention is scarcely convincing.

On firmer grounds lies the belief that Hans Christian Andersen was also a dyslexic. He was very behind-hand in his school work, being regarded at the time as a dullard. Even in later life he had never learned to spell correctly and his manuscripts reveal many errors of a type which are characteristic of dyslexia. Naturally enough these mistakes were usually detected and rectified by the publisher and printer.

TABLE IV. *From "H. C. Andersen og Charles Dickens" by E. Bredsdorff. Copenhagen 1951*

Manschester	Nord Kent Railrood	Brackfest	Schakspeare
Reventlau	Lindoa	Gioffry	Sidny Schmidt
Davistock	Davidstock	Lungh	Rodindendron
Mont Bank	Tamps	Temps	Punsch
Russel Place	Saturdai	Ierrold	Citty
Marry	Roschester	Khatedral	Henrik
Bulwor	Stroh	Cap	Schackspear
Lunz	Lung	Crismas Carols	Houscholds Word
Mackbeth	Machbeth	Stanfjeld	

Errors in spelling taken from Hans Christian Andersen's diary of his visit to London in 1857. With acknowledgements to Dr. Knud Hermann.

Occasionally, however, they escaped notice. Thus when Hans Christian Andersen wrote an account of his visit to Charles Dickens in London, names of English persons and places were often rendered incorrectly. These shortcomings were not always identified by his editors, so that they appeared in their original form in print (see Table IV).

Another retarded reader, possibly a dyslexic, was the Prince Imperial, son of Napoleon III. His tutors experienced great difficulty in teaching him to read and to write, though he was highly accomplished at sketching. Figure 36 shows a letter written by the Prince in 1863, when he was 7 years old, to General Bazaine, congratulating him on the capture of Puebla. In my possession there is the actual "reading machine" which was constructed for the Prince Imperial, and which was used by him at his lessons (see Frontispiece).

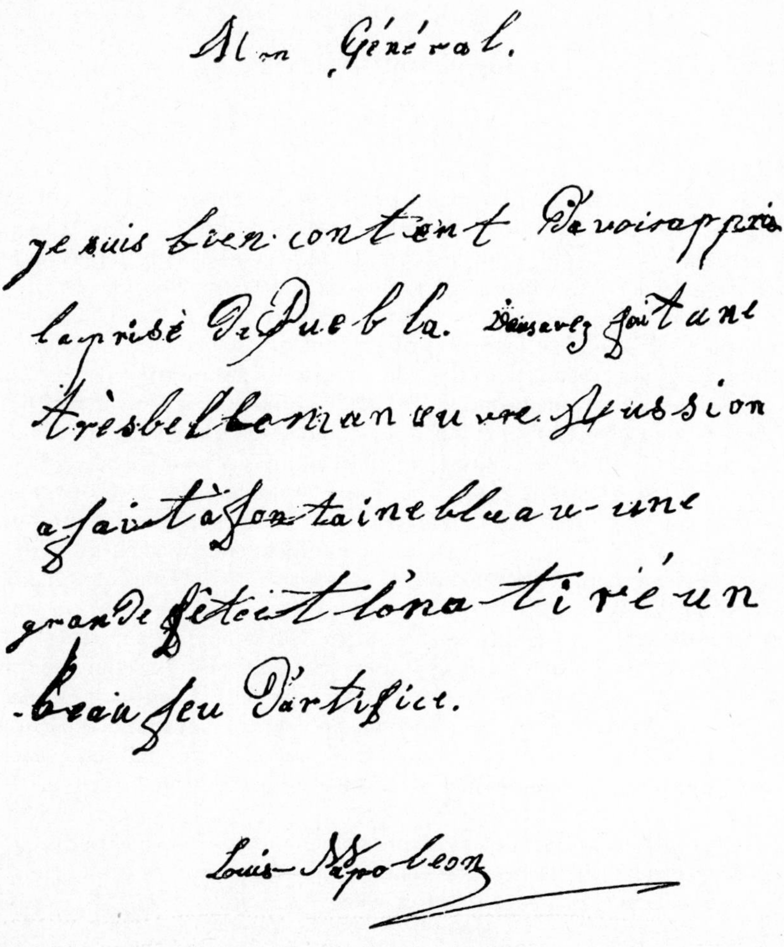
Mon Général.

je suis bien content de voir appris la prise de Puebla. Vous avez fait une très belle manœuvre. Russion a fait à Fontainebleau une grande fête et l'on a tiré un beau feu d'artifice.

Louis Napoleon

Fig. 36 Letter from the Prince Imperial to General Bazaine, written at the age of 7 (from *Le Prince Impérial*, by le Comte d'Herisson. Paris: Ollendorff, 1890, p. 85).

Chapter XIII
The nature of developmental dyslexia

We may attempt to sum up the opinions held currently by neurologists upon the topic of inherent reading difficulty in children. The problem is a big one and a complex one, for the total population of slow readers, retarded readers and poor readers, illiterates and semi-illiterates, is heterogeneous. Thus Monroe has spoken of a "constellation of factors in dyslexia", but perhaps it is more a question of a constellation of subtypes. Any total series will probably include some children who are dullards, if not indeed defectives. A number of brain-injured may find themselves within this broad group, the trauma dating from either pre- or post-natal life. There may also be included instances of neurological disease, not of traumatic nature, where reading is conspicuously difficult to learn. The pigeon-hole may be found to contain cases of disturbed or neurotic children whose emotional difficulties preclude learning. Educational progress may perhaps be handicapped by such unfavourable environmental circumstances as separation of parents, inconsistency of schooling, absenteeism through illness, delayed—or possibly even premature—attempts at teaching. The inherent nature of the language in question may play some part in bringing the reading defect to the notice of teachers at a very early stage. Even such physical factors as refractive errors or ocular imbalance may handicap some children in their attempts to read, while inconsistent manual preference may impose still further hardship upon them when they try to write.

But all the foregoing are epiphenomena. As we have already said, neurologists believe that in the heart of the community of poor readers there is a small hard core of cases where the tendency to the learning defect is inborn and independent of any intellectual inadequacies, emotional factors, educational or linguistic shortcomings which may happen to co-exist. Such are the cases which neurologists speak of as examples of specific, or developmental dyslexia. How large the problem is cannot be confidently stated, in the absence of large-scale surveys of retarded readers, with a satisfactory analytic breakdown by neurologists and their team of ancillary experts.

To identify these cases of specific developmental dyslexia among the multitude of poor readers is no easy task. A wide experience is demanded of the diagnostician, together with a freedom from prejudice. Even so the isolation is still a difficult matter, for there is no single clinical feature which can be accepted as pathognomic. Diagnosis requires a battery of tests and a knowledge of the patient's family circumstances, his personality, and his environment. In other words, there must be an appraisal of a veritable formula of findings embracing positive as well as negative issues.

Many hypotheses have been mooted to "explain" specific dyslexia. The earlier observers were struck by the resemblance of their cases with the phenomena of aphasic alexia from acquired disease. An agenesis of the cortex—especially in the region of one or both angular gyri—was often invoked. As long ago as 1906, Clairborne envisaged an "imperfect development and tardy reaction of the word- and letter-memory cells", high in the cerebral cortex, probably in the region of the left angular gyrus. Twenty years later, E. Bosworth McCready was inclined to regard dyslexic cases as being due to ontogenetic causes—a biological variation or stigma of degeneration, similar to colour-blindness and defective ocular fusion sense. Later still the author modified his views, believing that birth-trauma might be important.

Many such speculations are of mere historical interest.

Orton's theory of visual rivalry from inadequate unilateral occipital suppression is on the face of it too speculative to be acceptable. This idea does not explain why dimensions should be confused in a lateral direction only. Nor does it give any reason why verbal symbol-arrangement alone is at fault, while surrounding objects, scenes and pictures appear in normal orientation.

Any theory of minimal brain damage—whether or not sustained *in utero*—is also unconvincing. In the first place it conflicts with the factor of inheritance. It does not explain those cases where neurological deficits cannot be demonstrated even after the most searching techniques. Furthermore, the plasticity of the nervous system in the young might be expected to compensate for the effects of any circumscribed lesion of very early appearance. No brain-pathology has indeed ever been demonstrated in a case of developmental dyslexia, though this is an argument of lesser weight, for there is a striking absence of any autopsy material at all in cases of this kind.

Some writers have been tempted to look upon developmental dyslexia as not altogether a "specific" entity, but merely one aspect of inadequate achievement of the faculty of language. Thus, a form of congenital "aphasia" has been envisaged comparable with the disabilities which may follow acquired disease of the brain. As we have seen, these analogies have been stressed from the earliest days of our knowledge and are illustrated in the original term "congenital word-blindness". Just as modern aphasiologists look askance at any belief in pure or isolated dyslexia in adult cases, so too some writers insist that closer investigation of developmental dyslexics will always uncover other defects of a linguistic order. In particular, motor impairments of speech have been stressed. Whether these be simply articulatory in character, or whether they lie at a deeper level within the realm of language, or both, is not always made clear. Thus Monroe, who was impressed by the frequency of deviant speech in poor readers, thought that the two were causally related. Inaccurate diction, she said, might cause a confusion of sounds to be associated with the printed symbol. A child who has an articulatory defect hears the word as spoken by others in one way, and as spoken by himself, in another. Eisenson (1958) also drew attention to the possible detriment of faulty articulation upon learning, in that errors of pronunciation may cause errors in the interpretation of printed words. The child's concern over his way of talking may detract from his concentration upon the act of reading, and so lead to inadequate understanding. Furthermore, speech disorders, especially stuttering, may disturb the rate and rhythm of speaking, impair proper phrasing, and interfere with the comprehension of written symbols.

But there are weighty objections to the concept of developmental dyslexia as a fragment of congenital "aphasia". The idea is a specious one which must be scrutinised with caution. In the first place we know very little about the nature of the so-called congenital "aphasias". It would be better to speak merely of a comparison with cases of loss of language in the adult or older child, and not to try and exalt an analogy to the status of a hypothesis. The analogy has a certain utilitarian merit, but no more. There are profound differences, psychological, linguistic and philosophical, between the problem of a developmental dyslexic, and that of an adult who has long ago acquired language in the usual way and then lost it. The latter has been using it as a communicative tool for so many years that he has developed his own individual associations and has unwittingly built up a veritable idiolect. His vocabulary—available as well as practical—is rich, extensive and replete with memory-traces. The linguistic armamentarium may even include patterns from other cultures, as well as certain non-verbal systems of communication. Language has thus grown to be an integral part of his personality, and his use of language has become a highly specific aspect of his total behaviour. In such a person, circumscribed brain disease may impair this complex patterning, but the effect will bear only a superficial resemblance to the child who is slow in achieving this same faculty. Actually there is a vast difference between the problem of a mature and possibly scholarly adult who, as the result of a brain-lesion, finds it difficult by sweeping his gaze quickly over a line of print to utilise critical details and contextual analogies so as to identify the meaning of the text in the rough. At times even individual morphemes, words or phrases cannot be interpreted. The acquired dyslexic shares with the developmental dyslexic a greater or lesser lack of facility in the full appreciation of certain verbal symbols; but there the likeness rests, and the analogy should not be pressed further.

An acquired dyslexic may furthermore retain his ability to write fairly well. More often, however, he also finds it hard to express his ideas on paper, and to draw upon what was previously a very rich vocabulary, without betraying hesitancies repetitions, omissions and corrections. The graphic efforts of a child with developmental dyslexia are fundamentally different, and resemblances between the two kinds of dysgraphia will not stand up to scrutiny.

It is still necessary to emphasise these points despite the fact that they were clearly stated as long ago as 1903 at the Société de Neurologie de Paris, when R. Foerster presented the case of an imbecile who could not read. In the discussion which ensued, the topic was raised of illiteracy among children. Mme. Dejerine stressed that it was important not to confuse the pathological loss of a function with cases of absence of that function. Pierre Marie agreed, and went on to assert, "je ne crois pas que les troubles de la lecture observés chez nos malades soient en rien comparables à ceux de l'aphasie vraie".

The contemporary theory of cerebral immaturity, or maturational lag, demands serious attention. A developmental dyslexic is often regarded in American parlance as a "late bloomer", but only in regard to the flowering of certain specific faculties. The frequent occurrence of cortical equipotentiality—or rather, the lack of distinct unilateral cerebral dominance—is often adduced as supporting evidence. Electro-encephalographic data may also be quoted as being consonant with a state of cortical immaturity. L. Bender was one of the first to propound this theory, which she pleaded with eloquence. She regarded the notion as being based on a concept of functional areas of the brain and of personality which develop in a congenital fashion according to a recognised pattern. A maturational lag signifies a slow differentiation within this pattern. It does not imply a structural defect, deficiency, or loss. There is not necessarily any limitation in the potentialities, and, at variable levels, maturation may tend to accelerate, but often unevenly. These cases are understandable in terms of "embryonic plasticity"; i.e. being as yet unformed, but capable of being formed, being impressionable and responsive to patterning, carrying within themselves the potentialities of patterns which have not yet become fixed.

This attractive hypothesis raises its own train of questions. If specific developmental dyslexia represents a peculiar type of cerebral immaturity, it follows that the difficulty in reading might eventually improve—provided, of course, that attempts to learn are continued long enough. More information is needed here. Developmental dyslexia is certainly not often diagnosed in adulthood even though genuine instances are occasionally encountered, and the question naturally arises why this should be so. Perhaps the patient and his parents have resigned themselves to a state of hopeless ineducability, and no longer importune doctors and teachers. Perhaps the victims have merged into the amorphous population of adult illiterates and semi-illiterates.

Perhaps they have eventually made a degree of improvement so that they now achieve modest social and economic adjustment, but remain poor spellers, unwilling correspondents, and reluctant readers. Finally, it is conceivable that these childhood dyslexics—these slow bloomers— eventually mature, and blossom, so as no longer to be conspicuously handicapped.

Reference has already been made to the belief that some of these dyslexics eventually surmount their disability so as to achieve success and even distinction in adulthood. Hans Christian Andersen has already been quoted as such a late bloomer in the aptitude of reading. He is known to have been a very poor scholar, especially weak at reading and arithmetic, and never to have mastered the art of spelling. The manuscripts of his works betray numerous errors of a type which strongly suggests a dyslexic background. Being written in Danish these literary shortcomings probably elude all except Scandinavian students. In 1857, however, Andersen visited England. The diary of that visit was later published. Presumably the proof-reader corrected the more obvious mis-spellings, but he seems to have overlooked the inaccurate rendering of many proper names and English phrases, so that even to-day they appear in print in the original unorthodox form (see Table IV).

Obviously a large-scale longitudinal study or follow-up is needed of patients in whom the diagnosis of developmental dyslexia has been made in childhood by experienced neurologists.

The second problem which emerges from this hypothesis of maturational lag concerns the precise faculties which may be deemed to be concerned in the cases of dyslexia. It is hard to avoid the conclusion that mere visual non-identification of verbal symbols is not the whole story. Not only is it a matter of defective perception, but it is also one of inadequate association of lexical percepts. Clearly there is a tie-up between the recognition of the form of a visual symbol, and its acoustic properties. This process of linking one percept with another is where the principal fault may lie. As Vernon has emphasised, there is in reading-retardation a failure in analysis, abstraction and generalisation, one which is typically confined to linguistics. The cerebral activity which lags behind in maturation may be a specific cognitive act in which verbal symbols, auditory as well as visual, fail to achieve identity.

Obviously an auditory component is also concerned in the pathogenesis of dyslexia, as Fildes showed years ago, and as A. Bronner previously foreshadowed. Marshall and Ferguson (1939) spoke of a "difficulty" in remembering the mental picture of a word, though general memory is excellent . . . "(the dyslexic) just can't see meanings unless he can hear the word". The same writers spoke of dyslexia in terms of a sensori-motor integrative disability at the highest, or "skill" level. . . . The word-blind are limited chiefly by their inability to circumvent the visual speech associations, by acoustic as well as other channels.

J. Money (1962) has surmised that the dyslexic, in his difficulty in establishing lexical concepts, visual and auditory, may be of a non-visile cognitional type. Maybe he is weak in visual imagery and visual memory—the opposite of a person with eidetic imagery and photographic memory.

At an earlier date P. Schilder expressed some of these ideas in a more elaborate fashion. He traced the basic difficulty to an inability to differentiate the spoken word into its sounds, and to put the sounds together so as to constitute a word. Words and single sounds are brought into connection with a written word and a written letter, but these cannot be integrated and differentiated. This may be seen when a dyslexic, shown the word "banana" for instance, fails to grasp its meaning. Directed to spell it aloud, letter by letter, the dyslexic may correctly proclaim "B.A.N.A.N.A." but still be quite unable either to understand the word or to pronounce it. Schilder also referred to the common occurrence of mirror mistakes, and errors in the optic perception of letters. Dyslexia, he said, was an isolated trouble within a gnostic-intellectual function.

The rôle of maturational lag in developmental dyslexia has been elaborated somewhat by Birch (1962). From a conception of perceptual levels, Birch believes that a normal child passes through the stages, first of discrimination, then analysis, and later still synthesis. This perceptual development is sensitive to brain damage. One of the problems which contribute to a reading disability is the inadequate achievement of the higher and more complex levels of visual perceptual function. Birch has predicted that among those with reading disability one ought to be able to identify cases with very defective analytic and synthetic visual perceptual capacity. An additional or complementary hypothesis also discussed by Birch conceives of a hierarchy among the sensory systems. It is essential for reading readiness that the visual system should become dominant. Children who possess a different type of sensory protocol, make up a type with reading disability. The evolution of behaviour can be "conceptualised" as the process of development of intersensory patterning. Some victims of reading disability have impaired equivalences between the sensory systems. Birch believes that most children with reading disabilities find it difficult to establish visual-auditory equivalences, and perhaps visual-kinæsthetic and visual-tactual-kinæsthetic relations as well. His experimental findings support this belief, and he is of the opinion that his way of looking upon the problem of dyslexia offers the prospect of bringing to light important mechanisms.

To a clinical neurologist certain functions are recalled which are commonly regarded as being parieto-occipital in character. The not infrequent conjunction of dyslexia with directional disorders and with spatial defects, both of a personal and an extra-personal nature, may be cited as telling evidence. In so far as symbolic thinking is at fault, it is the parieto-occipital region of the dominant hemisphere which is under suspicion, that is if one can discern cerebral dominance at all in these dyslexic patients.

There are some who, looking behind the maturational inadequacy, seek to invoke a basic defect in Gestalt recognition. Visuo-verbal comprehension is naturally impaired. The spatial defects, reversals in reading and in writing, mixed hand-eye preferences, and other defects which may be met with in dyslexics are, according to A. L. Drew (1956), "variant manifestations in the fundamental defect in correct figure-ground recognition". Drew believed that "the inconsistencies, confusion, and apparently diametrically opposed findings reported in the literature and observed clinically can best be resolved by interpreting the findings in a configurational setting".

The adoption of some such theory of late blooming in a specific sense leads on to the question whether other specialised instances of maturational lag are ever encountered in neuro-pædiatric practice, which could be cited. A possible analogy with congenital auditory imperception, and also with congenital apraxia immediately comes to mind. Children with colour-blindness, lack of musical sense, deficient mathematical ability are more questionable analogues, for these short-comings are permanent rather than transient, and a maturational lag seems a scarcely tenable explanation here.

Does a specific cerebral immaturity imply a structural lesion, recognisable by present-day techniques? Probably not, though the question still cannot be answered with complete confidence. Certain contributors would appear from their writings to infer that some form of brain pathology, traumatic or otherwise, lies at the foundation of the pathogenesis of dyslexia, whether it be regarded as a dyssymbolia, or a maturational lag. The lack of autopsy data is a regrettable hiatus in our knowledge of developmental dyslexia. Even though it seems unlikely that any tangible evidence will emerge, it is clearly desirable that pathological studies should be made and published on children who have been earlier diagnosed as instances of developmental dyslexia. We recall that in the case of congenital auditory imperception, post-mortem study proved to be entirely negative in so far as cerebral pathology is concerned.

Chapter XIV
The dyslexic child grows up

That dyslexics are totally incapable of learning to read is a fallacy which seems to have been promulgated originally by Cyril Burt, and thereafter widely to have been accepted among educationalists. Neurologists do not agree with this *non possumus* viewpoint and have explicitly said so since the days of Hinshelwood (1917). Admittedly the prognosis may be more serious in developmental dyslexics than in cases of psychogenic reading retardation, but the outlook is anything but hopeless. With appropriate tuition dyslexics can make considerable progress and they may attain sufficient ability to read for all practical purposes. That is to say they become able to interpret notices, advertisements, newsprint and letters, but they will probably remain recalcitrant slow readers. Many ex-dyslexics, as they might be termed, perhaps never became "bookish" and may but rarely peruse a novel or magazine as a form of recreation, and for the sheer fun of it.

However, in the absence of organised skilled instruction, dyslexics are usually left to fend for themselves. Many of them drift—in an educational sense—and simply become items within the community of illiterates or near-illiterates. As such they will be barred from any lucrative or worthwhile profession and they will have to be content with work of a manual or practical kind. The victim may be rated fortunate if he does not swell the ranks of the delinquent or the antisocial.

The two following case-reports illustrate the type of niche into which a stable and not unintelligent dyslexic will fit, in the absence of specific tuition:

> P. M., male, aged 31 years, was never able to learn to read though good at most other subjects, and indeed top of the school in handicrafts. He left school at the age of 14 and served with the R.A.F. for 2 years. There he constantly confused right and left on the parade ground: he was unable to learn the Morse code for signalling purposes. His officer used to write his letters for him. He made close friends with another airman who was also dyslexic. On his return to civilian life he took a job as a dental mechanic which he held for 7 years. During that time he was able to memorise and recall the dental formulæ of all his employer's patients. He could drive a car well and comprehend the wayside road signs and traffic signals. Although unable to read a map fully, or to understand the sign-posts, he was able to motor all over England without getting lost. Similarly he could usually identify the individual discs in his collection of gramophone records.

On Raven's progressive matrices he scored 32 out of 60: his I.Q. was estimated to be 93. No neurological abnormality could be demonstrated but his ocular movements during the act of attempting to read were found by appropriate test-methods to be very abnormal (see Fig. 32). An E.E.G. revealed no pathological rhythms.

L. G., a coloured female aged 21 years was the youngest of five children. She attended a primary school in Trinidad but could never master the art of reading and was bottom in her class in this subject and also in spelling and writing to dictation. At arithmetic, history and English she was rated as average. This inability to read was a source of great distress to her and on leaving school at the age of 16 years she went to work with the express intention of saving enough money to go to England to learn to read. After 4 years she had accumulated sufficient for her fare. On her own initiative and without the help of friends or relatives in the Caribbean or in England she took passage in a ship and came to live and work in London, where she knew no one. She secured a job in a factory as a rag sorter and then sought help from her doctor as to her reading disability. Although unable to read she could find her way around London by comparing the number or destination of a bus with a pencilled note which a neighbour had given her. When shopping she would match the graphic symbols on the packages with those on her shopping list. Confronted with a printed word she might at times identify and read aloud correctly the constituent letters without, however, being able to name or to recognise the meaning of the word as a whole.

In other respects the patient was perfectly normal and no neurological abnormality could be detected. Her writing to dictation is shown in Fig. 20. The formal intelligence quotient was given as 65, but this was certainly a serious underestimate due to lack of cultural rapport with the psychometrist.

Arrangements were made for this patient to be employed in the hospital as a ward maid (where she proved highly efficient) and for her to receive tuition in reading at the hands of the Chaplain (no facilities being available within the sphere of the Ministry of Education).

In exceptionally auspicious circumstances, a dyslexic may fare better as he grows older, even though unassisted. This fact has been touched upon in the previous chapter. Given a good intellectual level, constancy of purpose, emotional stability and drive, the dyslexic may in later life manage to achieve such a modicum of literacy as to enable him to occupy a modest niche within the wage-earning community. He may even be lucky enough to benefit from some coaching at the hands of a sympathetic even if untrained teacher. Provided that the tuition is individual and intensive a partial success may reward unskilled or semi-skilled instruction at the hands of someone like a retired school-teacher or a parson.

In the next three cases, family circumstances were probably instrumental in securing for the dyslexic a better adjustment in adulthood.

J. P., male aged 33 years, had always experienced difficulty in learning to read. His two daughters were also retarded readers. In other respects his scholastic achievements were at least of average level. He attended a public school of an unorthodox sort, and then went to an Agricultural College. He managed to pass the first two examinations (out of a possible three) and in his studies he relied entirely upon lectures and demonstrations—text-books being impracticable. The patient now runs his own farm with complete success. Reading is managed with extreme slowness but he can cope with the ordinary circulars and news-headings. On reading aloud he was found to fare better with the longer nouns, verbs and adjectives, while frequently he would stumble over the short monosyllabic words, such as the articles, conjunctions and prepositions. His handwriting was neat but barely legible, and many odd errors in spelling were to be seen.

M. M., female aged 21 years, had attended an ordinary infant school, and from the start she experienced difficulty in learning to read. At first she was deemed to be lazy. Later she was suspected as being in need of glasses and these were ordered. She then went to a primary school, to a private school and finally finished at a secondary modern school, leaving at the age of 16 years. It was only when she went to a convent school in Singapore that something unusual was realised to be the matter with her. At no time did she see anyone from the Ministry of Education, although she was examined in a routine fashion by school medical officers, who "did not seem very interested". She sat her 11-plus examination, but failed because she could not read the test papers. When she left school she worked at a nursery crêche, and then she trained as a nurse for 2 years. She had to give this up, for the sister-tutor could never read her lecture-notes. She then spent a year among handicapped children, and now she is a nursing auxiliary at a mental hospital.

The difficulty in reading has persisted although she has mastered her defect up to a point; that is to say she can now read to the extent of beginning to look at books for her own pleasure though it takes her a very long time. She prefers magazines and short stories. From the start she found script more difficult than print and she could not consistently identify the ownership of various specimens of writing. She could always recognise numerals, but she was never very good at arithmetic. She can read traffic signs in the street, and she can follow T.V. and the cinema—except foreign films where she cannot fathom the English sub-titles which are exposed for too short a period of time. Rarely does she venture upon cross-word puzzles. She does not know whether she would be able to cope with musical notation, because her mother would never let her learn the piano.

At the age of 13 she went to Singapore—her father being a Naval Officer—and whilst there she learned to recognise a few of the more common Chinese symbols displayed in the streets.

Even today the patient's handwriting is very bad and barely legible, with frequent spelling mistakes of an unusual character (see Figs. 16, 17, 18). Certain characters are at times written in an unorthodox fashion. Sometimes two adjacent letters are not joined together; on other occasions they may be connected in a most unusual manner. Capital letters are sometimes incongruously interpolated and dots may be replaced by dashes. Occasionally she reverses a short word, as for example "if" which she writes as "fi". Finally, strange mistakes in spelling are often made involving not only long words, but also short words which should be familiar.

The patient declared herself to be right-handed, but she wore her wrist-watch on the right arm like many sinistrals do, and she folded her arms in a typical left-handed fashion. She stated that at one time she used to muddle up hopelessly her right and her left.

A.C., female aged 18 years, a member of a dyslexic family, had herself been severely retarded in learning to read. By dint of great application coupled with a background of high intelligence, she had largely mastered her disability though she never learned to spell correctly. A brilliant musical executant, she was considerably handicapped at the Royal College of Music because of her persistent inability to read musical notation.

In such a category too may belong the case of Karl XI (1655–97) who has been judged "one of Sweden's wisest kings". Succeeding to the throne at the age of 4 years he proved to be a most unsatisfactory scholar, mainly because of his inability to learn to read. His studies were supervised by Edmund Gripenhielm, Professor of History at the University of Uppsala. The monarch's progress in reading was extraordinarily slow and in adult life he always relied upon personal interviews rather than a study of reports. If handed a document he might be seen to hold the page upside-down and to pretend that he was reading the text. Throughout his life his spelling was highly unorthodox, the errors being quite unlike the usual mis-spellings of the uneducated. He would reverse words, omit letters, or start with letters belonging to the middle of a word. Perusal of his journals and *aides-mémoire* brings to light a number of startling mistakes; e.g. "ta" for "att"; "faton" for "aftou"; "wathen" for "staden"; "aagt" for "gott"; "årrgdh" for "gård"; "kråken" for "klockan"; "nathet" for "natten"; "tu" for "tva"; "byggninshielp" for "byggnadshjalp"; and "recyteran" for "rekryter". Reversals and other such spelling mistakes were habitual with him up to the time of his death.

Obviously it is most unsatisfactory that dyslexics should remain neglected as well as unrecognised; or that they should be allowed merely to muddle through as best they can. The disability is one which is amenable to treatment provided this be carried out with sufficient intensity, patience, sympathy and understanding. Perhaps, indeed, these qualities are more necessary to the teacher than any special pedagogic trick of technique or skill. The system of teaching adopted may matter less than the manner in which the instruction is imparted.

P. Sharp expressed this well when he wrote . . . "More important . . . than the training itself . . . is the quality of the teacher. Given the basic background and knowledge required to the handling of remedial cases, there is no substitute in the teacher for personality, a degree of missionary spirit, versatility, the pedagogical flair, patience, understanding, and the courage of one's convictions. When we consider the nature of the language disability and the complexity of language learning, it seems to me obvious that there is no one remedial method yet evolved which can be offered to teachers on a silver platter" (1951).

Nevertheless it is hard to escape the conclusion that it is important to the dyslexic (and to the community) for his disability to be recognised for what it is: and for unpropitious ways and circumstances of teaching to be avoided in favour of more appropriate methods. The dyslexic child obviously should no longer be taught in a large class where he is apt to find himself a cynosure and a butt. His reading lessons must be held in private, and his reading material should be interesting, even stimulating in nature.

It is a moot point whether this educational regime should be carried out at special schools, or in ordinary schools by way of a special teacher. Thus, on the one hand it might be deemed best to establish a number of educational establishments, either residential or non-residential, which would cater exclusively for dyslexic children. The example of schools for the deaf, the blind, and the speech-retarded comes to mind immediately. Our ignorance of the exact size of the dyslexic problem makes it hard to gauge whether or not this plan would be unnecessarily extravagant.

The alternative would be to establish a corps of selected teachers, who have been trained in the specific educational techniques appropriate for the dyslexic. These could then serve as peripatetic specialist teachers who would cover the schools within a region, and who would cope with selected pupils in a quiet and encouraging environment. Obviously as a necessary preliminary to such an organisation a systematic diagnostic service would be necessary, whereby dyslexic children could be identified within the population of dullards, neurotics, and slow readers.

The Danish system of training dyslexics which was instituted in 1935–36, may be quoted, although obviously the problem may not be the same in all countries. In Hellerup, one of the suburbs of Copenhagen, a large private house has been converted into a non-residential "Ordblinde Institut". The school copes with 100 pupils, the children entering at the age of 9 or 10 years. The duration of training averages two years. The pupils live at home and travel to and from the school in State supplied transport. In the case of children who live outside Copenhagen, lodgings are found near the institution. Tuition continues for 5 hours a day, 6 days a week. The daily curriculum comprises reading and writing (2 hours); arithmetic (1 hour); singing, drawing or handicraft (1 hour); and some other subject (1 hour). The classes for reading and writing are made up of 3 pupils to a teacher: in the case of arithmetic, however, the class may include as many as 12.

The teachers at the Institute previously have undergone special post-graduate training (lasting 2 to 3 months) for which they receive an additional diploma.

Early cases of dyslexia are selected at the ordinary schools where the classes ordinarily comprise 30 to 35 children. Those children who prove to be slow at learning to read are first of all referred to a special "reading class" within the ordinary school, where the pupils number 16 to one teacher. If, while in this class, the child is suspected of being a true dyslexic, he is referred to a diagnostic centre in Copenhagen. There a decision is made whether the scholar should be sent to the Word-blind Institute.

Most word-blind children come under the auspices of the State, and pay no fees. However, if the parents so wish, the pupils can also attend the Institute in a private capacity, the fees being 135 Kr. a month (£6 15s. 0d.).

After ordinary school hours, extension classes are held on the Institute premises until 9 p.m., for the benefit of adolescents and adults whose prior education in reading had been neglected. Two hundred such adults usually attend. As a rule the tuition is free but pupils can also be accepted on a private basis, the fees being 25 Kr. (£1 5s. 0d.) a month, comprising 2 hours a week.

In addition to the Ordblinde Institut there is a continuation school (Hellerup-hus Efterskole) close by. This caters on a non-residential basis for those of 14 years of age or more who need further help with reading and writing. This course of instruction lasts one year and the curriculum comprises 6 hours a day. Ordinarily the State is responsible for the fees but here again private pupils may be accepted who pay 80 Kr. (£4) a month, for 6 to 8 hours a day.

The staff is made up of 40 teachers, 20 being full-time and 20 part-time, and the teachers are shared between the two institutes. In addition there exists in Denmark an official register of these specially trained teachers of the word-blind who will accept private patients.

Various specialised ways of teaching dyslexics have from time to time been advanced, e.g. the Norrie phonetic system, and the Borel-Maisonny gestural method. But an outsider may perhaps feel, as did Orton, that "anything that will work is a good method".

One may reproduce a table giving the end-results of a series of cases of dyslexia which have received training at the Ordblinde Institut. Hermann has set out the occupations held by ex-scholars, in correlation with their ages and the length of time after leaving the Institute.

The exact methods of teaching constitute a technical side of pedagogy which cannot be discussed in a work such as this. Certain general principles can, however, be stressed.

(1) The contemporary "look and say" method of reading should be replaced by a more phonic or analytic-synthetic system in the case of dyslexics.

(2) The progression from simple tasks to more complex ones should be made slowly and gradually.

(3) Visual learning should be reinforced by other sense-channels. Thus the dyslexic child should be taught to learn the appearances of a letter (or word); to say the symbol aloud; to trace its outlines digitally; and to write it down.

(4) The reading-material chosen for learning purposes should be interesting and exciting for the young reader.

(5) Toys, incorporating letters and words, should be encouraged as a sort of ancillary play-therapy.

(6) The teaching should be individual and intense. Here Monroe's figures for the results of treatment of children with retarded reading may be quoted; it must be recalled that Monroe did not accept the concept of dyslexia though her series must surely have included a number of such cases. Eighty-nine children who were poor readers received remedial training under close supervision: of these 93% made "accelerated progress" and 5% made normal progress. Of 50 children who received remedial instruction in reading, but at their own schools from their own teachers, 52% made accelerated progress and 14% made a normal progress. Of another 50 children who received no remedial instruction in reading at all, none made accelerated progress; 4% made normal progress; and 96% made "retarded progress".

TABLE V

PUPILS AND GRADUATES OF THE
COPENHAGEN WORD-BLIND INSTITUTE
(1935–36)

Total	Present Status	Born 1924 or earlier	Born 1925 –1929	Born 1930 –1934	Born 1935 or later
84	Still attending school	1	2	41	40
23	Passed entrance examination, Institute of Higher Education	—	1	2	2
	Students, I.H. Ed.	1	10	2	—
	Graduates, I.H. Ed.	1	4	—	—
16	Passed entrance examination, Teachers' College	—	—	1	2
	Students, Teachers' College	1	2	8	2
8	Kindergarten teachers	1	1	3	3
5	Other types of teacher-training	1	3	1	—
29	Student nurses	2	6	11	1
	Nurses	3	1	—	—
	Children's nurses	—	2	3	—
48	Shop assistants	1	2	3	—
	Trainees	2	3	18	14
	Higher executives	2	1	1	1
25	Clerical work Junior clerks	—	1	6	3
	Clerks	4	2	7	2
86	Skilled workers Apprentices	—	5	22	17
	Artisans	16	12	13	1
69	Unskilled workers Labourers	9	8	3	2
	Factory workers, storemen	4	6	6	2
	Mates and errand-boys	1	3	6	19
47	Domestic work Domestic helps	1	4	15	16
	Housewives	7	4	—	—
5	Journalism	3	—	2	—
17	Armed Forces Conscripts	—	2	9	1
	N.C.O.s and Officers	—	3	2	—
5	Fishermen	2	1	—	2
24	Agriculture	2	3	11	8
17	Other occupations	—	4	10	3
33	Unemployed	10	2	12	9
541		75	98	218	150

(After Hermann 1959)

(7) In order that the child may concentrate upon learning to read, write and spell, some subject or subjects may require to be sacrificed from the school curriculum. Thus it may well be considered more important for the dyslexic to lose his disability than to try and cope with some less essential subject such as Latin, French, or algebra.

(8) In uncomplicated cases of dyslexia, i.e. where no serious neurotic problem exists, psychological treatment is unnecessary or even perhaps unwise. Joss, Leiman and Schiffman (1961) have quoted an experimental series of 40 children with reading problems. They were divided into 4 groups of ten. One group received remedial reading and psychotherapy; one group was given remedial reading alone; a third received psychotherapy only; and the fourth group received no treatment at all. The results seemed—as far as they were reliable—to favour the rôle of remedial reading.

Bibliography

Åberg, A. (1958), *Karl XI*, Wahlstrom & Widstrand, Stockholm.

Alajouanine, Tn., Lhermitte, F., de Ribaucourt-Ducarne, B. (1960), Les Alexies agnosiques et aphasiques, in *Les Grandes Activités du Lobe Occipital*, Paris, Masson, p. 235.

Altus, G. T. (1956), A WISC Profile for Retarded Readers, *J. Consult. Psychol.*, **20**, 155–156.

Anderson, C. J., Merton, E. (1920), Remedial Work in Reading, *Elem. School J.*, **20**, 685–701, 772–791.

Anderson, I. H., Dearborn, W. F. (1952), *The Psychology of Teaching Reading*, New York, Ronald Press.

Anderson, M., Kelley, M. (1931), An Inquiry into Traits Associated with Reading Disability, *Smith College Stud. in Social Work*, **2**, 46–63.

Arthur, G. (1940), Therapy with Retarded Readers, *J. Consult. Psychol.*, **4**, 173–176.

Axline, V. M. (1947), Non-directive Therapy for Poor Readers, *J. Consult. Psychol.*, **11**, 61–69.

Bachmann, F. (1927), Uber kongenitale Wortblindheit (angeborene Leseschwäche), *Abhandl. Neur. Psych. Psychol. Grenzgeb.*, **40**, 1–72.

Bakwin, H. (1950), Psychiatric Aspects of Pediatrics: Lateral Dominance, Right- and Left-handedness, *J. Pediat.*, **36**, 385–391.

Barger, W. C., Lavin, R., Speight, F. S. (1957), Constitutional Psychiatry of Poor Readers, *Dis. Nerv. Sys.*, **18**, 289–294.

Bastian, H. C. (1898), *A Treatise on Aphasia and Other Speech Defects*, London, Lewis.

Bateman, F. (1890), *On Aphasia or Loss of Speech*, 2nd Edit., London, J. & A. Churchill.

Bender, L. (1956), Problems in Conceptualisation and Communication in Children with Developmental Alexia, *Proc. Amer. Psychobiol. Ass.*

Bender, L. (1956), Research Studies from Bellevue Hospital on Specific Reading Disabilities, *Bull. Orton Soc.*, **6**, 1–3.

Bender, L. (1957), Specific Reading Disability as a Maturational Lag, *Bull. Orton Soc.*, **7**, 9–18.

Bender, L. (1959), Report on Dyslexia—International Congress of Child Psychiatry, *Bull. Orton Soc.*, **9**, 26.

Bender, L., Schilder, P. (1951), Graphic Art as a Special Ability in Children with a Reading Disability, *J. clin. exp. Psychopath.*, **12**, 147–156.

Bennett, C. C. (1938), An Inquiry into the Genesis of Poor Reading, *Contrib. Educ. No. 755, Bureau Publ., Teaching Coll., Columbus Univ.*

Benton, A. L. (1958), Significance of Systematic Reversal in Right-left Discrimination, *Acta Psych. Neur. Scand.*, **33**, 129–137.

Benton, A. L. (1959), *Right-left Discrimination and Finger-localisation: Development and Pathology*, New York, Paul C. Hoeber.

Benton, A. L. (1962), Dyslexia in Relation to Form Perception and Directional Sense, Chap. VI of *Reading Disability. Progress and Research Needs in Dyslexia*, edit. J. Money. Baltimore, John Hopkins Press.

Benton, A. L., Kemble, J. D. (1960), Right-left Orientation and Reading Disability, *Psych. & Neur.*, **139**, 49–60.

Berkhan, O. (1885), Uber die Störung der Schriftsprache bei Halbidioten und ihre Ähnlichkeit mit den Stammeln, *Arch. f. Psych.*, **16**, 78–86.

Berkhan, O. (1917), Uber die Wortblindheit im Stammeln im Sprechen und Schreiben, ein Fehl im Lesen, *Neurol. Centralbl.*, **36**, 914–927.

Berlin, R. (1887), *Eine besondere Art der Wortblindheit (Dyslexia)*, Wiesbaden.

Betts, E. A. (1936), *The Prevention and Correction of Reading Difficulties*, San Francisco, Row.

Betts, E. A. (1950), *Foundations of Reading Instruction with Emphasis on Differentiated Guidance*, Amer. Book Co.

Birch, H. G. (1962), Dyslexia and the Maturation of Visual Function, Chap. X of *Reading Disability. Progress and Research Needs in Dyslexia*, edit. J. Money. Baltimore, John Hopkins Press.

Bjork, A. (1955), The Electromyogram of the Extraocular Muscles in Opticokinetic Nystagmus and in Reading, *Acta Ophth.*, **33**, 437–454.

Bladergroen, W. J. (1955), Uber die Diagnostik und Therapie von Lesehemmungen, *Prax. Kinderpsychol.*, **4**, 6–14.

Blanchard, P. (1936), Reading Disabilities in Relation to Difficulties of Personality and Emotional Development, *Ment. Hyg.*, **20**, 384–413.

Blanchard, P. (1946), Psychoanalytic Contributions to the Problems of Reading Disabilities, *Psychoanal. Stud. Child.*, **2**, 163–188.

Blom, E. C. (1928), Mirror Writing, *Psychol. Bull.*, **25**, 582–594.

Bond, G. L., Tinker, M. A. (1957), *Reading Difficulties, their Diagnosis and Correction*, New York, Appleton-Century-Crofts.

Borel-Maisonny, S. (1956), Dyslexie et dysorthographie, *Rev. franç. hyg. med. schol. univ.*, **9**, 15–24.

Boyce, E. R. (1949), *Learning to Read*, London, Macmillan.

Broadbent, W. (1872), Cerebral Mechanisms of Speech and Thought, *Trans. Roy. Med. Chir. Soc.*, **55**, 145–194.

Broadbent, W. (1896), Note on Dr. Hinshelwood's Communication on Word-blindness and Visual Memory, *Lancet*, **1**, 18.

Bronner, A. F. (1917), *The Psychology of Special Abilities and Disabilities*, Boston, Little, Brown & Co.

Burt, C. (1950), *The Backward Child*, 3rd Edit., London, Univ. Lond. Press.

Burt, C. (1960), The Readability of Type, *New Scientist*, **7**, 277–279.

Buswell, G. T. (1947), The Sub-vocalisation Factor in the Improvement of Reading, *Elem. School J.*, **48**, 190–196.

Carnvale, E. (1961), The Etiology of Reading Disability, *Lab. Rep. No. 2, Comm. Proj. Sect., Ment. Health Study Center.*

Carter, D. B. (1953), A Further Demonstration of Phi Movement in Cerebral Dominance, *J. Psychol.*, **36**, 299–309.

Carter, H. J. L. (1930), Disabilities in Reading, *Elem. School. J.*, **31**, 120–132.

Center, B. (1954), Perceptual Function in Reading Problems, *Optom. Weekly*, **45**, 311–312.

Chesni, Y. (1959), Retard de langage chez l'enfant. Recherche statistique sur la dyslexie specifique en relation avec les troubles de la dominance laterale et de l'orientation spatio-temporale, *Rev. neur.*, **101**, 576–582.

Childs, S. B. (1959), The Teaching of Reading Abroad, *Bull Orton Soc.*, **9**, 19–25.

Clairborne, J. H. (1906), Types of Congenital Symbol Amblyopia, *J. Amer. Med. Ass.*, **47**, 1813–1816.

Claparède (1916), Bradylexie bei einem sonst normalen Kinde, XI Meeting Swiss Neurol. Soc., May 13 and 14, *Abs. Neur. Zlbl.*, 1917, **36**, 572.

Clark, B. (1935), The Effect of Binocular Imbalance on the Behaviour of the Eyes During Reading, *J. Educ. Psychol.*, **26**, 530–538.

Clark, B. (1940), Binocular Anomalies and Reading Ability, *Am. J. Oph.*, **23**, 885–891.

Cohn, R. (1961), Delayed Acquisition of Reading and Writing Abilities in Children: a Neurological Study, *Arch. neur.*, **4**, 153–164.

Cole, E. M. (1942), The Neurologic Aspects of Defects in Speech and Reading, *New Eng. J. Med.*, **226**, 977–980.

Comfort, F. D. (1931), Lateral Dominance and Reading Disability, *Am. Psychol. Assoc.*, Sept. 11, 1931, Toronto.

Creak, M. (1936), Reading Difficulties in Children, II, *Arch. Dis. Child.*, 143–156.

Critchley, M. (1927), *Mirror Writing*, London, Kegan Paul.

Critchley, M. (1927), Some Defects of Reading and Writing in Children: Their Association with Word-blindness and Mirror-writing, *J. State med.*, **35**, 217–223.

Critchley, M. (1942), Aphasic Disorders of Signalling (Constitutional and Acquired) Occurring in Naval Signalmen, *J. Mount Sinai Hosp.*, **9**, 363–375.

Critchley, M. (1953), *The Parietal Lobes*, London, Arnold.

Critchley, M. (1961), Doyne Memorial Lecture, Inborn Reading Disorders of Central Origin, *Tr. Oph. Soc.*, **81**, 459–480.

Critchley, M. (1962), Developmental Dyslexia: a Constitutional Dyssymbolia, in *Word-blindness or Specific Developmental Dyslexia*, edit. A. W. Franklin. London, Pitman Med. Publ. Co. Ltd., pp. 45–48.

Critchley, M. (1963), The Problem of Developmental Dyslexia, *Proc. Roy. Soc. Med.*, **56**, 209–212.

Currier, F. P., Jr., Dewar, M. (1927), Word-blindness: Difficulty in Reading in School-children, *J. Mich. Med. Soc.*, **26**, 300–304.

Dale, N. (1902), *Further Notes on the Teaching of English Reading*, London and Liverpool, Philip & Son.

Daniels, J. C. (1962), Reading Difficulty and Aural Training, in *Word-blindness or Specific Developmental Dyslexia*, edit. A. W. Franklin. London, Pitman Med. Publ. Co. Ltd., pp. 87–92.

Daniels, J. C., Diack, H. (1956), *Progress in Reading*, Univ. Nottingham Inst. Educ.

Dearborn, W. F. (1931), Ocular and Manual Dominance in Dyslexia, Paper read before Amer. Psychol. Ass., Sept. 11, 1931, Toronto.

Dearborn, W. F. (1933), Structural Factors which Condition Special Disability in Reading, *Proc. 57th Ann. Sess., Amer. Ass. Ment. Def.*, p. 268.

Dearborn, W. F., Leverett, H. M. (1945), Visual Defects and Reading, *J. exp. Educ.*, **13**, 111–124.

Dejerine, J. (1892), Contribution à l'étude anatomo-pathologique et clinique des differents variétés de cecité verbale, *Comp. rend. scéan. soc. biol.*, sér. 9, **4**, 61–90.

Delacato, C. H. (1959), *The Treatment and Prevention of Reading Problems*, Springfield, Ill., C. C. Thomas.

Diack, Hunter (1960), *Reading and the Psychology of Perception*, Nottingham, Peter Skinner Publishing Ltd.

Dolch, E. W. (1948), *Problems in Reading*, Garrard Press.

Dosužkov, B. (1961), Vztak motorické a sensorické laterality u leváku, *Čžl. Neur.*, **24**, 136–143.

Downey, J. E. (1927), Types of Dextrality and their Implications, *Amer. J. Psychol.*, **38**, 317–367.

Drew, A. L. (1956), A Neurological Appraisal of Familial Congenital Word-blindness, *Brain*, **79**, 440–460.

Duche, J. (1958), Les dyslexies, *Rev. franç hyg. ment. scol.*, **11**, 129–138.

Dugas, M. (1956), Dyslexies et dysorthographies, *Presse méd.*, **64**, 1435–1438.

Duguid, K. (1935), Congenital Word-blindness and Reading Disability, *Guy's Hosp. Rep.*, **85**, 76–93.

Duncan, J. (1953), *Backwardness in Reading: Remedies and Prevention*, London, Harrap.

Durbrow, H. C. (1952), Teaching the Strephosymbolic. 1. At the Primary Level, *Bull. Orton Soc.*, **2**, 7–9.

Eames, T. H. (1932), A Comparison of the Ocular Characteristics of Unselected and Reading Disability Groups, *J. Educ. res.*, **25**, 211–215.

Eames, T. H. (1934), Low Fusion Convergence as a Factor in Reading Disability, *Am. J. Oph.*, **17**, 709–710.

Eames, T. H. (1935), A Frequency Study of Physical Handicaps in Reading Disability and Unselected Groups, *J. Educ. res.*, **29**, 1–5.

Eames, T. H. (1938), The Ocular Conditions of 350 Poor Readers, *J. Educ. res.*, **32**, 10–16.

Eames, T. H. (1944), Amblyopia in Cases of Reading Failure, *Am. J. Oph.*, **27**, 1374–1375.

Eames, T. H. (1945), Comparison of Childern of Premature and Full-term Birth who Fail in Reading, *J. Educ. res.*, **38**, 506–508.

Eames, T. H. (1948), Incidence of Diseases Among Reading Failures and Nonfailures, *J. Pediat.*, **33**, 614–617.

Eames, T. H. (1948), Comparison of Eye Conditions Among 1,000 Reading Failures, 500 Ophthalmic Patients, and 150 Unselected Children, *Am. J. Oph.*, **31**, 713–717.

Eames, T. H. (1955), The Relationship of Birth Weight, the Speeds of Object and Word Perception, and Visual Acuity, *J. Pediat.*, **47**, 603–606.

Edfeldt, A. W. (1959), *Silent Speech and Silent Reading*, Stockholm, Almqvist & Wiksell.

Ellis, A. (1949), Results of a Mental Hygiene Approach to Reading Disability Problems, *J. Consult. psychol.*, **13**, 56–61.

Engler, B. (1917), Über Analphabetia Partialis: (kongenitale Wortblindheit), *Monat. Psych. Neur.*, **42**, 119–132.

Ettlinger, G., Jackson, C. V. (1955), Organic Factors in Developmental Dyslexia, *Proc. Roy. Soc., Med.*, **48**, 998–1000.

Eustis, R. S. (1947), The Primary Etiology of the Specific Language Disabilities, *J. Pediat*, **31**, 448–455.

Eustis, R. S. (1947), Specific Reading Disability, *New Engl. J. Med.*, **237**, 243–249.

Ewart, E. (1955), A Reading Disability Analysed: Word-blindness, *The Schoolmaster*, 1073–1074.

Fabian, A. A. (1945), Vertical Rotation in Visual Motor Performance; its Relationship to Reading Reversals, *J. Educ. Psychol.*, **36**, 129–145.

Faust, C. (1954), Hirnpathologische Studie zur kongenitalen Schreib-Lese-Schwäche, *Nervenarzt.*, **4**, 137–145.

Fernald, G. (1943), *On Certain Language Disabilities: Nature and Treatment*, Baltimore, Williams & Wilkins.

Fernald, G., Keller, H. (1921), The Effect of Kinæsthetic Factors in the Development of Word-recognition in Non-readers, *J. Educ. res.*, **4**, 355–377.

Feyeux, A. (1932), *L'Acquisition du Langage et ses Retards*, Paris, Editions Médicales N. Maloine.

Filbin, R. L. (1957), Prescription for the Johnny Who Can't Read, *Elementary English*, **34**, 559–561.

Fildes, L. G. (1921), A Psychological Inquiry into the Nature of the Condition Known as Congenital Word-blindness, *Brain*, **44,**, 286–307.

Fisher, J. H. (1905), A Case of Congenital Word-blindness (Inability to Learn to Read), *Oph. Rev.*, **24**, 315–318.

Fisher, J. H. (1910), Congenital Word-blindness (Inability to Learn to Read), *Trans. Oph. Soc. U.K.*, **30**, 216–225.

Flesch, R. (1955), *Why Johnny Can't Read*, New York, Harper.

Foerster, R. (1904), A propos de la Pathologie de la Lecture et de l'Ecriture (cécité verbale congénitale chez un débile), *Rev. neur.*, **12**, 200–202.

Forgays, D. G. (1953). The Development of Differential Word Recognition. *J. exp. Psychol.*, **45**, 165–168.

Frank, H. (1936), "Word-blindness" in School-children, *Trans. Oph. Soc. U.K.*, **56**, 231–238.

Frank, H. (1935), A Comparative Study of Children who are Backward in Reading and Beginners in the Infant School, *Brit. J. Educ. psychol*, **5**, 41–58.

Franklin, A. W. (1962), Ed. *Word-blindness or Specific Developmental Dyslexia*, London, Pitman Med. Publ. Co. Ltd.

Franstrom, K. O. (1958), Difficulties in Reading and Writing (Word Blindness). III. Ophthalmological Aspects. *Nord. med.*, **59**, 518–519.

Freeman, F. N. (1916), Experiments with School-subjects: Observations of Eye-movements in Reading, *Experimental Education*, pp. 95–109, Houghton Mifflin Co.

Freeman, J. D. J. (1957). Reading Difficulties in Childhood, *Trans. oph. soc. U.K.*, **77**, 611–613.

Freud, S. (1953), *On Aphasia*, London, Imago Publ. Co. Trans. by E. Stengel. (Originally published 1891).

Gallagher, J. R. (1960), Specific Language Disability: Dyslexia, *Bull. Orton Soc.*, **10**, 5–10.

Gallagher, J. R. (1962), Word-blindness (Reading-disability; Dyslexia): Its Diagnosis and Treatment, in *Word-blindness or Specific Developmental Dyslexia*, edit. E. W. Franklin. London, Pitman Med. Publ. Co. Ltd., pp. 6–14.

Gann, E. (1945), *Reading Difficulty and Personality Organisation*, New York, Kings Crown Press, Columbia Univ.

Gates, A. I. (1922), The Psychology of Reading and Spelling with Special Reference to Disability, *Teachers Coll. Contrib. Educ. No.* 129. Teachers Coll., Columbia Univ.

Gates, A. I., Bond, G. L. (1936), Reading Readiness. A Study of Factors Determining Success and Failure in Beginning Reading, *Teach. Coll. Rec.*, **37**, 679–685.

Gates, A. I. (1937), Diagnosis and Treatment of Extreme Cases of Reading Disability, *Nat. Soc. Stud. Educ. Yearbook*, 36 (1), 391, Chicago.

Gates, A. I. (1941), The Role of Personality Maladjustment in Reading Disability, *J. genet. psych.*, **59**, 77–83.
Gates, A. I., Bond, G. L. (1936), Relation of Handedness, Eye-sighting and Acuity Dominance to Reading, *J. Educ. psychol.*, **27**, 450–456.
Geiger, R. (1923), A Study in Reading Diagnosis, *J. Educ. Res.*, **8**, 282–300.
Gellerman, S. W. (1949), Causal Factors in the Reading Difficulties of Elementary School-children, *Elem. School J.*, **49**, 523–530.
Gillingham, A. (1956), The Prevention of Scholastic Failure Due to Specific Language Disability, *Bull. Orton Soc.*, **6**, 26–31.
Gillingham, A., Stillman, B. U. (1956), *Remedial Training for Children with Specific Disability in Reading, Spelling, and Penmanship* (5th Edit.), New York, Sackett and Wilhelms Litho. Corp.
Gjessing, H. J. (1958), Reading Difficulties in Children, *T. norske Laegef.*, **78**, 187–191.
Goetzinger, C. P., Dirks, D. D., Baer, C. J. (1960), Auditory Discrimination and Visual Perception in Good and Poor Readers, *Ann. Otol. Rhin. Laryng.*, **69**, 121–136.
Goins, J. T. (1958), Visual Perceptual Abilities and Early Reading Progress, *Suppl. Educ. Monogr. No.* 87, Chicago.
Goldberg, H. K. (1959), The Ophthalmologist Looks at the Reading Problem, *Am. J. Oph.*, **47**, 67–74.
Goldberg, H. K., Marshall, C., Sims, E. (1960), The Role of Brain Damage in Congenital Dyslexia, *Am. J. Oph.*, **50**, 586–590.
Gooddy, W. (1963), Directional Features of Reading and Writing, *Proc. Roy. Soc. Med.*, **56**, 206–212.
Gooddy, W., Reinhold, M. (1961), Congenital Dyslexia and Asymmetry of Cerebral Function, *Brain*, **84**, 231–242.
Granjon-Galifret, N., Ajuriaguerra, J. (1951), Troubles de l'apprentissage de la lecture et dominance latérale, *Encéphale*, **40**, 385–398.
Granstrom, K. O., Åberg, A. (1961), Kunglig ordblindhet. Karl XI's läsochskrivsvårigheter, *Svenska Lakertidn.*, **58**, 915–927.
Gray, W. S. (1921), Diagnostic and Remedial Steps in Reading, *J. Educ. res.*, **4**, 1–15.
Gray, W. S. (1922), *Remedial Cases in Reading: Their Diagnosis and Treatment*, Suppl. Educ. Monogr. No. 22, Depart. Educ., Chicago Univ., Chicago Press.
Gray, W. S. (1956), *Teaching of Reading and Writing: An International Survey*, UNESCO monogr., Evans Bros. Ltd., London.
Grewel, F. (1958), Ontwikkelingsdyslexie (Leeszwakte), *Nederl. Tijd. Geneesk.*, 102. 183–190.
Gruber, E. (1962), Reading Ability, Binocular Coordination and the Ophthalmograph, *Arch. Oph.*, **67**, 280–288.
Günther, M. (1928), Beitrage zur Psycho-pathologie und Klinik der sogennanten kongenitalen Leseschwäche, *Ztschr. kinderforsch.*, **34**, 585.
Hall, R., Word-blindness: its Cause and Cure.
Hallgren, B. (1950), Specific Dyslexia, *Acta psych. neur.*, Suppl. No. 65, 1–287.
Hallgren, B. (1952), Specifik Dyslexi, *Socialmed. Tidskr.*, **29**, 70–78.
Hambright, H. (1956), The Prevention of Scholastic Failure Due to Specific Language Disability, *Bull. Orton Soc.*, **6**, 32–36.
Hardy, W. G. (1962), Dyslexia in Relation to Diagnostic Methodology in Hearing and Speech Disorders, in *Reading Disability*, edit. J. Money. Baltimore, John Hopkins Press.
Harris, A. J. (1957), Lateral Dominance, Directional Confusion and Reading Disability, *J. Psychol.*, **44**, 283–294.
Harris, A. J., Roswell, F. G. (1953), Clinical Diagnosis of Reading Disability, *J. Psychol.*, **36**, 323–340.
Hawthorne, J. W. (1935), The Effect of Improvement in Reading Ability on Intelligence Test-scores, *J. Educ. Psychol.*, **26**, 41–51.
Heller, T. M. (1963), Word-blindness; a Survey of the Literature and a Report of Twenty-eight Cases, *Pediatrics*, **31**, 669–691.
Henry, S. (1947), Children's Audiograms in Relation to Reading Attainments, *J. genet. Psychol.*, **70**, 211–231; **71**, 3–48; 49–63.

Hermann, K. (1949), Alexia-agraphia. A Case Report (Acquired Reading and Writing Disabilities, Temporary Word-blindness of the Congenital Type), *Acta psych. neur.*, **25**, 449–455.

Hermann, K. (1956), Congenital Word-blindness, *Acta Psych. Neur. Scand.*, Suppl. 108, 117–184.

Hermann, K. (1959), *Reading Disability*, Copenhagen, Munksgaard.

Hermann, K. (1961), Kliniske Iagttagelser und medfødt ordblindhed, *Nord. Tidssk. for Tale og Stemme*, **21**, 31–40.

Hermann, K., Norrie, E. (1958), Is Congenital Word-blindness a Hereditary Type of Gerstmann's Syndrome? *Psych. Neur.*, **136**, 59–73.

Hermann, K. and Voldby, H. (1946), The Morphology of Handwriting in Congenital Word-blindness, *Acta Psych. Neur.*, **21**, 349–363.

Hibbert, F. G. (1961), Dyslexia, Proc. Soc. Brit. Neurosurg., 62nd Meeting at Swansea, Nov. 25–26, 1960. Reported in *J. Neur. Neurosurg. Psych.*, 1961, **24**, N.S. 93–94.

Hildreth, G. (1936), *Learning the Three Rs*, Minneapolis Educ. Publ., pp. IX and 824.

Hildreth, G. (1945), A School Survey of Eye-hand Dominance, *J. Appl. Psychol.*, **29**, 83–88.

Hilman, H. H. (1956), The Effect of Laterality on Reading Disability, *Durham Res. Rev.*, **7**, 86–96.

Hincks, E. (1926), *Disability in Reading in Relation to Personality*, Harvard Monogr. Educ., Whole No. 7, Ser. 1, Vol. 2, No. 2, Camb. Univ. Press.

Hinshelwood, J. (1895), Word-blindness and Visual Memory, *Lancet*, **2**, 1564–1570.

Hinshelwood, J. (1896), A Case of Dyslexia: a Peculiar Form of Word-blindness, *Lancet*, **2**, 1451–1454.

Hinshelwood, J. (1896), The Visual Memory for Words and Figures, *Brit. med. J.*, **2**, 1543–1544.

Hinshelwood, J. (1898), A Case of "Word" without "Letter" Blindness, *Lancet*, **1**, 422–425.

Hinshelwood, J. (1899), "Letter" without "Word" Blindness, *Lancet*, **1**, 83–86.

Hinshelwood, J. (1900), Congenital Word-blindness, *Lancet*, **1**, 1506–1508.

Hinshelwood, J. (1900), *Letter-, Word- and Mind-blindness*, London, Lewis.

Hinshelwood, J. (1902), Four Cases of Word-blindness, *Lancet*, **1**, 358–363.

Hinshelwood, J. (1902), Congenital Word-blindness, with Reports of Two Cases, *Oph. Rev.*, **21**, 91–99.

Hinshelwood, J. (1904), A Case of Congenital Word-blindness, *Ophthalmoscope*, **2**, 399–405.

Hinshelwood, J. (1904), A Case of Congenital Word-blindness, *Brit. med. J.*, **2**, 1303–1307.

Hinshelwood, J. (1907), Four Cases of Congenital Word-blindness Occurring in the Same Family, *Brit. med. J.*, **2**, 1229.

Hinshelwood, J. (1911), Two Cases of Hereditary Word-blindness, *Brit. med. J.*, **1**, 608.

Hinshelwood, J. (1912), The Treatment of Word-blindness, Acquired and Congenital, *Brit. med. J.*, **2**, 1033–1035.

Hinshelwood, J. (1917), *Congenital Word-blindness*, London, Lewis.

Hirsch, K. de (1957), Tests Designed to Discover Potential Reading Difficulties at the 6-year-old Level, *Amer. J. Orthopsych.*, **27**, 566–576.

Hoffmann, J. (1927), Uber Entwicklung und Stand der Lesepsychologie, *Arch. ges. Psychol.*, **57**, 401–444.

Hoffmann, J. (1927), Experimentalpsychologische Untersuchungen über Leseleistungen von Schulkinden, *Arch. ges. Psychol.*, **58**, 325–388.

Holt, L. M. (1962), The Treatment of Word-blind Children at Saint Bartholomew's, in *Word-blindness or Specific Developmental Dyslexia*, edit. A. W. Franklin. London, Pitman Med. Publ. Co. Ltd., pp. 93–98.

Holt, M. (1963), Children Suffering from Word Blindness, *A.W.B.C. Bulletin*, **1**, 3–4.

Huey, E. B. (1908), *The Psychology and Pegagogy of Reading*, New York, Macmillan Co.

Illing, E. (1929), Uber kongenitale Wortblindheit (angeborene Schreib- und Leseschwäche), *Monat. Psych. Neur.*, **71**, 297–355.

Ingram, T. T. S. (1959), Specific Developmental Disorders of Speech in Childhood, *Brain*, **82**, 450–467.

Ingram, T. T. S. (1959), A Description and Classification of the Common Disorders of Speech in Children, *Arch. Dis. Child.*, **34**, 444.

Ingram, T. T. S. (1960), Pædiatric Aspects of Specific Developmental Dysphasia, Dyslexia and Dysgraphia, *Cerebral Palsy Bull.*, **2**, 254–277.

Ingram, T. T. S. (1963), The Association of Speech Retardation and Educational Difficulties, *Proc. Roy. Soc. Med.*, **56**, 199–203.

Ingram, T. T. S., Reid, J. F. (1956), Developmental Aphasia Observed in a Department of Child Psychiatry, *Arch. Dis. Child.*, **31**, 161–172.

Jackson, E. (1906), Developmental Alexia (Congenital Word-blindness), *Amer. J. med. Sci.*, **131**, 843–849.

Jackson, J. (1944), A Survey of Psychological, Social and Environmental Differences between Advanced and Retarded Readers, *J. genet. Psychol.*, **65**, 113–131.

Jansky, J. J. (1958), A Case of Severe Dyslexia with Aphasic-like Symptoms, *Bull. Orton Soc.*, **8**, 8–10.

Jastak, J. (1934), Interferences in Reading, *Psychol. Bull.*, **31**, 244–272.

Jenkins, D. L., Brown, A. W., Elmendorf, L. (1937), Mixed Dominance and Reading Disability, *Amer. J. Orthopsych.*, **7**, 72–81.

Jones, M. M. W. (1944), Relationship between Reading Deficiencies and Left-handedness, *School & Soc.*, **60**, 238.

Judd, C. H., Buswell, G. T., *Silent Reading: A Study of Various Types*, Suppl. Educ. Monogr., Dept. Educ., Univ. Chicago, No. 23.

Judd, C. H., Gray, W. S., McLaughlin, K., Schmidt, C., Gilliland, A. R. (1918), *Reading: Its Nature and Development*, Suppl. Educ. Monogr., Dept. Educ., Univ. Chicago II, No. 4.

Kabersek, V. (1960), *L'Electro-oculographie ou l'enregistrement des mouvements oculaires. Son application à l'etude de la lecture normale et des anomalies pathologiques de la Lecture*, Paris, Foulon.

Kågén, B. (1943), Om ordblindhet, *Pedagog. skrifter.*, **60**, 179–180.

Kawi, A. A., Pasamanick, B. (1958), Association of Factors of Pregancy with Reading Disorders in Childhood, *J. Amer. Med. Assoc.*, **166**, 1420–1423.

Kawi, A. A., Pasamanick, B. (1959), Prenatal and Paranatal Factors in the Development of Childhood Reading Disorders, *Monogr. Soc. Res. Child. Dev.*, **24**, No. 4, 1–80.

Kennard, M. A., Rabinovitch, R. D., Wexler, D. (1952), The Abnormal Electroencephalogram as Related to Reading Disability in Children with Disorders of Behavior, *Canad. Med. Ass. J.*, **67**, 330–333.

Kerr, J. (1897), School Hygiene, in its Mental, Moral and Physical Aspects. Howard Medal Prize Essay, *J. Roy. Statist. Soc.*, **60**, 613–680.

Kerr, J. (1900), Four Unusual Cases of Sensory Aphasia, *Lancet*, **1**, 1446.

Kirmsse (1917–18), Die Priorität in der Begriffsbildung "Wortblindheit", *Zeit. Kinderforsch.*

Krabbe, M. J. (1954), Word-blindness and Image Thinking, *Acta psychother.*, **2**, 52–64.

Krise, E. M. (1949), Reversals in Reading: a Problem in Space Perception, *Elem. School J.*, **49**, 278–284.

Krise, E. M. (1952), An Experimental Investigation of Theories of Reversals in Reading, *J. Educ. Psychol.*, **43**, 408–422.

Kurk, M., Steinbaum, M. (1957), Factors in Reading Disability, *Rev. Optom.*, **94**, 25–26.

Kuromaru, S. and Okada, S. (1961), On Developmental Dyslexia in Japan, Paper read at the 7th Internat. Congr. Neurol., Rome.

Lachmann, F. M. (1960), Perceptical-motor Development in Children Retarded in Reading-ability, *J. Consult. Psychol.*, **24**, 427–431.

Langman, M. P. (1960), The Reading Process: a Descriptive, Interdisciplinary Approach, *Genet Psychol. Monogr.*, **62**, 3–40.

Larmande, A., Sutter, J. M. (1954), Dissociation des acuités visuelles et dyslexie spécifique, *Bull. Soc. franç. Ophth.*, **67**, 220–225.

Larsen, C. Å. (1954), Huad er ordblindhed. In: *2 nord. staevne for laesepaedegogen*, p. 73.

Laubenthal, F. (1936), Uber "kongenitale Wortblindheit", zugleich ein Beitrag zur Klinik sog. partieller Schwächsinnsformen und ihrer erblichen Frundlagen, *Zeit. Neur. Psych.*, **156**, 329–360.

Laubenthal, F. (1938), Uber einige Sonderformen des "angeborenen Schwächsinns" (klinischer und erbbiologischer Beitrag zur Kenntnis der kongenitalen Wortblindheit und Worttaubheit, der Hörstörungen bei Schwächsinnigen und der xeroder mischen Idiotie), *Zeit. Neur. Psych.*, **163**, 233–288.

Laubenthal, F. (1941), Zur Erbhygienischen Bewertung der kongenitalen Wortblindheit, *Der Erbarzt.*, **9**, 156.

Launay, C. (1952), Etude d'une classe d'enfants de 6 à 7 ans inaptes à la lecture, *Sem. Hôp. Paris*, **28**, 1459–1463.

Launay, C. (1952), Etude d'ensemble des inaptitudes à la lecture, *Sem. Hôp. Paris*, **28**, 1463–1474.

Launay, C., Borel-Maisonny, S. (1952), Un cas de "dyslexie spécifique", *Sem. Hôp. Paris*, **28**, 1455–1459.

Lefevre, C. A. (1961), Reading Instruction Related to Primary Language Learning: a Linguistic View, *J. devel. Reading*, **4**, 147–158.

Lewis, H. W., Jr. (1961), A Study of Reading Levels: Standardised Tests and Informal Tests, The Reading Clinic, Publ. Schools Dist., Columbia.

Ley, A. (1938), Sur l'alexie d'évolution familiale et héréditaire, *Ann. med.-psychol.* **96**, (II), 145–150.

Ley, J., Tordeur, G. W. (1936), Alexie et agraphie d'évolution chez des jumeaux monozygotiques, *J. belge neur. psych.*, **36**, 203–222.

Liessens, P. (1949), L'alexie chez les enfants arriérés, *Acta neur. psych. belg.*, **49**, 102–112.

Looft, C. (1939), Dyslexi og dysgrafi hos skolebarn, *Nord. med.*, **3**, 2621–2626.

Lord, E. E., Carmichael, L., Dearborn, W. F. (1925), *Special Disabilities in Learning to Read and Write*, Harv. Monogr. Educ., Whole No. 6, Ser. 1, Vol. 2, No. 1, Camb. Univ. Press.

Lynn, R. (1955), Personality Factors in Reading Achievement, *Proc. Roy. Soc. Med.*, **48**, 996–997.

Lynn, R. (1957), Temperamental Characteristics Related to Disparity of Attainment in Reading and Arithmetic, *Brit. J. educ. Psychol.*, **27**, 62–67.

Mach, L. (1937), Lese-und Schreibschwäche bei normalbegabten Kindern, *Zeit. Kinderforsch.*, **46**, 113–197.

Macmeeken, A. M. (1939), *The Intelligence of a Representative Group of Scottish Children*, London, Univ. Lond. Press.

Macmeeken, A. M. (1939), *Ocular Dominance in Relation to Developmental Aphasia*, London, Univ. Lond. Press.

Malmquist, E. (1958), *Factors Relating to Reading Disabilities in the First Grade*, Stockholm, Almqvist & Wiksell.

Margolin, J. B., Roman, M., Harari, C. (1955), Reading Disability in the Delinquent Child: a Microcosm of Psychological Pathology, *Am. J. Orthopsych.*, **25**, 25–35.

Mark, H. J., Hardy, W. G. (1958), Orienting Reflex Disturbances in Central Auditory or Language Handicapped Children, *J. Speech Hear. Dis.*, **23**, 237–242.

Marshall, W., Ferguson, J. H. (1939), Hereditary Word-blindness as a Defect of Selective Association, *J. Nerv. Ment. Dis.*, **89**, 164–173.

Maruyama, M. (1958), Reading Disability: a Neurological Point of View, *Bull. Orton Soc.*, **8**, 14–16.

Mayer, K. (1928), Uber kongenitale Wortblindheit, *Monat. Psych. Neur.*, **70**, 161–177.

McCready, E. B. (1909–10), Congenital Word-blindness as a Cause of Backwardness in School-children: Report of a Case Associated with Stuttering, *Penn. med. J.*, **13**, 278–284.

McCready, E. B. (1926–27), Defects in the Zone of Language (Word-deafness and Word-blindness) and their Influence in Education and Behaviour, *Am. J. Psych.*, **6** (O.S. **83**), 267–277.

Meredith, C. P. (1963). The Association for Word Blind Children, *A.W.B.C. Bulletin*, **1**, 1–2.

Meredith, P. (1962), Psycho-physical Aspects of Word-blindness and Kindred Disorders, in *Word-blindness or Specific Developmental Dyslexia*, ed. A. W. Franklin. London, Pitman Med. Publ. Co. Ltd., pp. 28–40.

Meyer, H. (1937), Laesevanskeligheder Los Børn (Ordblindhed), *Vor Ungdom.*, **59**, 253.

Miles, T. R. (1962), A Suggested Method of Treatment for Specific Dyslexia, in *Word-blindness or Specific Developmental Dyslexia*, ed. A. W. Franklin. London, Pitman Med. Publ. Co. Ltd., pp. 99–104.

Miles, T. R. (1963). Comments on the Report on "Dyslexia" published in the *Health of the School Child, 1962. A.W.B.C. Bulletin*, **1**, 2–3.

Miller, A. D., Margolin, J. B., Yolles, B. F. (1957), Epidemiology of Reading Disabilities: Some Methodologic Considerations and Early Findings, *Amer. J. Publ. Health*, **47**, 1250–1256.

Ministry of Education (1956), Pamphlet No. 30, *Education of the Handicapped Pupil 1945–1955*, London, H.M.S.O., p. 26. (Reprinted 1960.)

Ministry of Education (1957), Pamphlet No. 32, *Standards of Reading 1948–1956*, London, H.M.S.O., p. 46.

Ministry of Education (1962), *The Health of the School Child*, London, H.M.S.O., p. 248.

Money, J. (1962), Ed. *Reading Disability. Progress and Research Needs in Dyslexia*, Baltimore, John Hopkins Press.

Monroe, M. (1932), *Children Who Cannot Read*, Chicago, Univ. Chicago Press.

Monroe, M., Backus, B. (1937), *Remedial Reading*, Boston, Houghton Mifflin.

Moor, L. (1961), L'examen psychologique chez les dyslexiques et les dysorthographiques, *Med. Infant.*, **68**, 43–47.

Morgan, D. H. (1939), Twin Similarities in Photographic Measures of Eye-movements while Reading Prose, *J. Educ. Psychol.*, **30**, 572–586.

Morgan, W. Pringle (1896), A Case of Congenital Word-blindness, *Brit. med. J.*, **2**, 1378.

Mosse, H. L., Daniels, C. R. (1959), Linear Dyslexia. A New Form of Reading Disorder, *Amer. J. Psychother.*, **13**, 826–841.

Muller, R. G. E. (1960), Die visuelle Erfassung von Buchstaben bei legasthenischen Schulkindern, *Psychol. Beitr.*, **5**, 416–427.

Nadoleczny, M. (1913), Uber die Unfähigkeit lesen zu lernen (sogenannte kongenitale Wortblindheit) und ihre Beziehung zu Sprachstörungen, *Monat. Kinderh.*, **12** (Referate) 336–340.

Namnum, A., Prelinger, E. (1961), On the Psychology of the Reading Process, *Amer. J. Orthopsych.*, **31**, 820–828.

Nettleship, E. (1901), Cases of Congenital Word-blindness (Inability to Learn to Read), *Ophthal. Rev.*, **20**, 61–67.

Newbrough, J. R., Kelly, J. G. (1962), A Study of Reading Achievement in a Population of School-children, in *Reading Disability*, ed. J. Money. Baltimore, John Hopkins Press, pp. 61–72

Nicholls, J. V. V. (1959), The Office Management of Patients with Reading Difficulties, *Canad. Med. Assoc. J.*, **81**, 356–360.

Nicholls, J. V. V. (1960), Congenital Dyslexia: a Problem in Aetiology, *Canad. med. ass. J.*, **82**, 575–579.

Norrie, E. (1939), *Om Ordblindhed*, Copenhagen.

Norrie, E. (1951), Ord-, tal- og nodenblindhed. Musikpaedagogen.

Norrie, E. (1954), Ordblindhedens (dyslexiens) arvegang, *Laesepaedagogen*, **2**, 61.

Ombredane, A. (1937), Le mechanisme et la correction des difficultés de la lecture connues sous le nom de cecité verbale congénitale, *Rapp. Psych. Schol. ler. Cong. Psych. Inf.*, Paris, 201–233.

Opitz, R. (1913), Einige Fälle von Wortblindheit, *Arch. Pädogog.*, **2**, 79.

Orton, J. L. (1957), The Orton Story, *Bull. Orton Soc.*, **7**, 5–8.

Orton, S. T. (1925), Word-blindness' in School-children, *Arch. neur. psych.*, **14**, 581–615.

Orton, S. T. (1928), Specific Reading Disability—Strephosymbolia, *J. Amer. Med. Ass.*, **90**, 1095–1099.

Orton, S. T. (1928), An Impediment in Learning to Read—a Neurological Explanation of the Reading Disability, *School & Soc.*, 286–290.

Orton, S. T. (1934), Some Studies in Language Function, *Res. Publ. Ass. Res. Nerv. Ment. Dis.*, **13**, 614–633.
Orton, S. T. (1937), *Reading, Writing and Speech Problems in Children*, London, Chapman & Hall.
Orton, S. T. (1943), Visual Functions in Strephosymbolia, *Arch. Ophth.*, **30**, 707–717.
O'Sullivan, M. A., Pryles, C. U. (1962), Reading Disability in Children, *J. Pediat.*, **60**, 360–375.
Park, G. E. (1953), Mirror and Reversed Reading, *J. Pediat.*, **42**, 120–128.
Park, G. E. (1959), Medical Aspects of Reading Failures in Intelligent Children, *Sight-sav. Rev.*, **29**, 213–218.
Peters, A. (1908), Uber kongenitale Wortblindheit, *Munch. med. Woch.*, **55**, 1116 and 1239.
Peters, W. (1926), Psychologische Untersuchungen über Lesedefekte, *Zeit. Pädagog. Psychol.*, **27**, 31–45.
Petty, L. (1960), A Normative Study of Reading Difficulty in Delinquents, *Delaware St. med. J.*, **32**, 24–26.
Petty, M. C. (1939), An Experimental Study of Certain Factors Influencing Reading Readiness, *J. Educ. Psychol.*, **30**, 215–230.
Pflugfelder, G. (1948), Psychologische Analyse eines Fall von angeborener Lese- u. Schreibschwäche, *Monat. Psych. Neur.*, **115**, 55–79.
Pintner, R. (1913), Inner Speech During Silent Reading, *Psychol. Rev.*, **20**, 129–157.
Plate, E. (1909), Vier Fälle von kongenitaler Wortblindheit in einer Familie, *Münch. med. Woch.*, **56**, 1793.
Prechtl, H. F. R. (1962), Reading Difficulties as a Neurological Problem in Childhood, in *Reading Disability*, ed. J. Money. Baltimore, John Hopkins Press, pp. 187–193.
Prechtl, H. F. R., Stemmer, J. C. (1959), Ein choreatiformes Syndrom bei Kindern, *Wien. med. Woch.*, **109**, 461–463.
Prechtl, H. F. R., Stemmer, J. C. (1962), The Choreiform Syndrome in Children, *Dev. Med. Child Neur.*, **4**, 119–127.
Pritchard, E. (1911), Intermittent Word-blindness, *The Ophthalmosc.*, **9**, 171–172.
Rabinovitch, R. D. (1959), Reading and Learning Disabilities, being Chap. 43 in *Amer. Handb. Psych.*, Edit. Arieti, Vol. 1, Basic Books Inc., New York, pp. 857–869.
Rabinovitch, R. D. (1962), Dyslexia: Psychiatric Considerations, in *Reading Disability*, ed. J. Money. Baltimore, John Hopkins Press.
Rabinovitch, R. D., Drew, A. L., De Jong, R. N., Ingram, W., Withey, L. (1954), A Research Approach to Reading Retardation, in Neurology and Psychiatry in Childhood, *Res. Publ. Ass. nerv. ment. Dis.*, **34**, 363–396.
Rabkin, J. (1956), Reading Disability in Children, *S. Afr. med. J.*, **30**, 678–681.
Ranschburg, P. (1916), Die Leseschwäche (Legasthenie) und Rechenschwäche (Arithemie), der Kinder im Lichte des Experiments, *Abh. aus. d. Grenzgeb. Päd. Med., Berlin*.
Ranschburg, P. (1925), Psychopathologie der Störungen des Lesens, Schreibens und Rechnens im Schulkindesalter, *Ber. uber d. 2, Kongr. Heilpäd im Munchen*, Springer, Berlin.
Ranschburg, P. (1927), Zur Pathophysiologie der Sprech-, Lese-, Schreib- und Druckfehler, *Psych. neur. Woch.*, **29**, 19–20.
Ranschburg, P. (1928), *Die Lese- u. Schreibstörungen des Kindesalters*, Halle, Marhold.
Reinhold, M. (1962), The Diagnosis of Congenital Dyslexia, in *Word-blindness or Specific Developmental Dyslexia*, ed. E. W. Franklin. London, Pitman Med. Publ. Co. Ltd., pp. 70–73.
Reinhold, M. (1963), The Effect of Laterality on Reading and Writing, *Proc. Roy. Soc. Med.*, **56**, 203–206.
Rémond, A., Gabersek, V. (1956), Lunettes pour l'enregistrement des électro-oculogrammes, *Rev. neur.*, **94**, 847–848.
Rémond, A., Gabersek, V. (1956), Technique et méthode d'enregistrement des mouvements des yeux en clinique neurologique. Application à l'étude de la lecture, *Rev. neur.*, **95**, 506–509.
Rémond, A., Gabersek, V. (1956), Les cheminements du regard au cours de la lecture. I. Les mouvements des yeux, *Rev. neur.*, **95**, 510–516.

Rémond, A., Gabersek, V. (1956), Les cheminements du regard au cours de la lecture. II. Les stations du regard, *Rev. neur.*, **95**, 516–521.

Rémond, A., Gabersek, V., Lesèvre, N. (1956), Corps d'oeil sur l'efficacité du regard dans la lecture, *Rev. neur.*, **95**, 455–470.

Rémond, A., Lesèvre, N., Gabersek, V. (1957), Approche d'une sémeiologie électrographique du regard, *Rev. neur.*, **96**, 536–546.

Riis-Vestergaard, I. (1962), Treatment at the Word-blind Institute, Copenhagen, in *Word-blindness or Specific Developmental Dyslexia*, ed. E. W. Franklin. London, Pitman Med. Publ. Co. Ltd., pp. 15–22.

Robinson, H. (1937), The Study of Disabilities in *Elem. School* Reading, *J.*, **38**, 1–14.

Robinson, H. M. (1946), *Why Pupils Fail in Reading*, Chicago, Univ. Chic. Press.

Rønne, H. (1936), Congenital Word-blindness in School-children, *Tr. Oph. Soc. U.K.*, **56**, 311–333.

Rønne, H. (1937), Medfødte Laesevanskligheder hos Skolebørn, *Ugesk. f. Laeger*, **9**, 185–192.

Rønne, H. (1943), Medicinske og paedagogiske problemer i ordblindesagen, *Social-paedagog. tidsskr.*, **3**, 121.

Rosenberg, M. E. (1961), A Brief Look at the State of Reading Retardation, *Labor Rep. No.* 1, *Commun. Projects Sect., Ment. Health Study Center.*

Roundinesco, Trélat, J. (1950), Note sur la dyslexie, *Bull. Soc. méd. Hôp. Paris*, **66**, 1451–1458.

Runge, (1926), Uber die sogenannt. kongenitale Wortblindheit, *Zlbl. Neur. Psych.*, **42**, 813–814.

Rutherfurd, W. J. (1909), The Aetiology of Congenital Word-blindness, with an Example, *Brit. J. Child. Dis.*, **6**, 484–488.

Schilder, P. (1944), Congenital Alexia and its Relation to Optic Perception, *J. genet. psychol.*, **65**, 67–88.

Schiøler, E. (1952), Ordblindhed-lidt om diagnose og undervisningsmetoder, *Paedagog.-psykolog. tidskr.*, **12**, 24.

Schlossman, A. (1960), Reading Difficulties in Children, *Eye, Ear, Nose, Thr. Monthly*, **39**, 514–518.

Schmitt, C. (1918), Developmental Alexia, *Elem. School J.*, **18**, 680–700.

Schonell, F. J. (1945), *The Psychology of Teaching Reading*, Edinburgh and London, Oliver & Boyd.

Schonell, F. J. (1948), *Backwardness in the Basic Subjects*, 4th Edit., Edinburgh and London, Oliver & Boyd.

Schrock, R. (1912), Uber kongenitale Wortblindheit, Rats-u. Univ. Buchdruckerei Adlers Erben Rostock.

Schwalbe-Hansen, P. A. (1937), Om "Ordblinde" Børn, *Ugesk. f. Lager.*, **99**, 520–522.

de Séchelles (1962), The Treatment of Word-blindness, in *Word-blindness or Specific Developmental Dyslexia*, ed. E. W. Franklin. London, Pitman Med. Publ. Co. Ltd., pp. 23–27.

Sédan, J. (1951), Arithmo-alexie congénitale, *Rev. d'oto-neuro-ophtal.*, **23**, 118–120.

Seymour, P. J. (1959), Efficient Reading, *Amer. orthop. J.*, **9**, 73–76.

Shankweiler, D. P. (1962), Some Critical Issues Concerning Developmental Dyslexia, in *Word-blindness or Specific Developmental Dyslexia*, ed. E. W. Franklin. London, Pitman Med. Publ. Co. Ltd., pp. 51–55.

Sharp, P. (1956), Teaching the Strephosymbolie at the High School Level, *Bull. Orton Soc.*, **6**, 20–22.

Sheldon, W., Hubble, D. V. (1960–61), Educational Problems in Children, *Trans. Hunterian Soc.*, **19**, 106–128.

Shepherd, E. M. (1956), Reading Efficiency of 809 Average School-children. *Amer. J. Oph.*, **41**, 1029–1039.

Silver, A. A., Hagin, R. (1960), Specific Reading Disability: Delineation of the Syndrome and Relationship to Cerebral Dominance, *Compreh. psych.*, **1**, 126–134.

Sinclair, A. H. (1948), Developmental Aphasia, *Brit. J. Ophth.*, **32**, 522–531.

Skydsgaard, H. B. (1942), *Den konstitutionelle dyslexi*, Copenhagen.

Bibliography 101

Skydsgaard, H. B. (1944), Dyslexiens prognose, *Skolehyg. tidskr.*
Smith, D. E. P., Carrigan, P. M. (1959), *The Nature of Reading Disability*, New York, Harcourt, Brace & Co.
Solms, H. (1947), Beitrag zur Lehre von der sog. kongenitalen Wortblindheit, *Monat. Psych. Neur.*, **115**, 1–54.
Spiel, W. (1953), Beitrag zur kongenitalen Lese- und Schreibstörung, *Wien. Zeit. Nervenh. u. Grenzgeb.*, **7**, 20–35.
Statten, T. (1953), Behaviour Patterns, Reading Disabilities, and EEG Findings, *Amer. J. Psych.*, **110**, 205–206.
Steen, S. W. (1958), Lesevansker hos barn og øyeundersøkelse av barn, *T. norske Laegeforen.*, **78**, 186–187.
Stephenson, S. (1907), Six Cases of Congenital Word-blindness Affecting Three Generations of One Family, *The Ophthalmoscope*, **5**, 482–484.
Stewart, R. E. (1950), Personality Maladjustment and Reading Achievement, *Amer. J. Orthopsych.*, **20**, 410–417.
Subirana, A., Corominas, J., Oller-Daurel a L. (1950), Las Afasias congenitas infantiles, *Actas Luso-esp. neur. psiq.*, **9**, 14–25.
Sutherland, A. H. (1922), Correcting School Disabilities in Reading, *Elem. School J.*, **23**, 37–42.
Tamm, A. (1924), Undersokningar av i skolan efterblivna barn, *Hygeia*, **86**, 673–706.
Tamm, A. (1927), Medfödd ordblindhet och därmed besläktade rubbningar i barnaaldern, *Svenska läk.-sällsk. handl.*, **53**, 143–155.
Tamm, A. (1927), Die angeborene Wortblindheit und verwandte Störungen bei Kindern, *Zeit. psychoanal. Pädagog.*, **1**, 329.
Tamm, A. (1943), Ordblindhet hos barn, *Pedagog. skr.*, **5**, 179–180.
Taylor, E. A. (1957), The Spans: Perception, Apprehension and Recognition, *Amer. J. Ophth.*, **44**, 501–507.
Thomas, C. J. (1905), Congenital Word-blindness and its Treatment, *Ophthalmoscope*, **3**, 380–385.
Thomas, C. J. (1908), The Aphasias of Childhood and Educational Hygiene, *Publ. Health*, **21**, 90–100.
Thompson, L. J. (1956), Specific Reading Disability—Strephosymbolia. 1. Diagnosis, *Bull. Orton Soc.*, **6**, 3–9.
Tjossem, T. D., Hansen, T. J., Ripley, H. S. (1962), An Investigation of Reading Difficulty in Young Children, *Amer. J. Psychiat.*, **118**, 1104–1113.
Variot, G., Lecomte (1906), Un cas de typhbolexie congénitale (cécité congénitale verbale, *Gaz. Hôp.*, **79**, 1479–1481.
Vermeylen, G. (1930), Un trouble rare de l'evolution du langage chez un enfant de 8 ans, 10 *Cong. belge neur. psych. J. de Neur.*, **30**, 827–836.
Vernon, M. D. (1957), *Backwardness in Reading. A Study of its Nature and Origin*, Cambridge, Camb. Univ. Press.
Wall, W. D. (1945), Reading Backwardness Among Men in the Army (1), *Brit. J. Educ. Psych.*, **15**, 28–40.
Wall, W. D. (1946), Reading Backwardness Among Men in the Army (2), *Brit. J. Educ. Psych.*, **16**, 133–148.
Wallin, J. E. H. (1921), Congenital Word-blindness, *Lancet*, **1**, 890–892.
Walter, K. (1954), Beitrag zum Problem der angeborenen Schreib- Lese- Schwache, (Kongenitale Wortblindheit), *Nervenarzt.*, **25**, 146–154.
Walters, R. H., van Loan, M., Crofts, J. (1961), A Study of Reading Disability, *J. cons. Psych.*, **25**, 277–283.
Warburg, F. (1911), Uber die angeborene Wortblindheit und die Bedeutung ihrer Kenntines fur den Unterricht, *Zeit. Kinderforsch.*, **16**, 97.
Wawrik, M. (1931), Eine experimentell-psychologische Untersuchung uber zwei Falle von Leseschwäche, *Zeit. Kinderforsch.*, **38**, 462–515.
Witty, P. A., Kopel, D. (1936), Sinistral and Mixed Manual Ocular Behaviour in Reading Disability, *J. Educ. Psychol.*, **27**, 119–134.
Witty, P. A., Kopel, D. (1936), Factors Associated with the Etiology of Reading Disability, *J. Educ. Psychol.*, **27**, 222–230.
Witty, P. A., Kopel, D. (1936), Heterophoria and Reading Disability, *J. Educ. Psych.*, **27**, 222–230.

Witty, P. A., Kopel, D. (1936), Studies of Eye-muscle Imbalance and Poor Fusion in Reading Disability, *J. Educ. Psych.*, **27**, 663–671.

Wolfe, L. (1941), Differential Factors in Specific Reading Disability. (1) Laterality of Functions, *J. Genet. Psych.*, **58**, 45–56.

Wolff, G. (1916), Uber kongenitale Wortblindheit, *Cor. -Bl. f. schweiz. Ärzte*, **46**, 237–238.

Wollnerr, M. H. B. (1958), Some European Research in Reading Disabilities, *Education*, **78**, 555–560.

Woody, C., Phillips, A. J. (1934), The Effects of Handedness on Reversals in Reading, *J. Educ. Res.*, **27**, 651–662.

Yedinack, J. G. (1949), A Study of the Linguistic Functioning of Children with Articulation and Reading Disabilities, *J. Genet. Psych.*, **74**, 23–59.

Zangwill, O. L. (1960), *Cerebral Dominance and its Relation to Psychological Function*, Edinburgh, Oliver & Boyd.

Zenner (1893), Ein Fall von Unfähigheit zu Lesen (Alexie), *Neur. Zlbl.*, **12**, 293–299.

Index